Hypertension and Stress
A Unified Concept

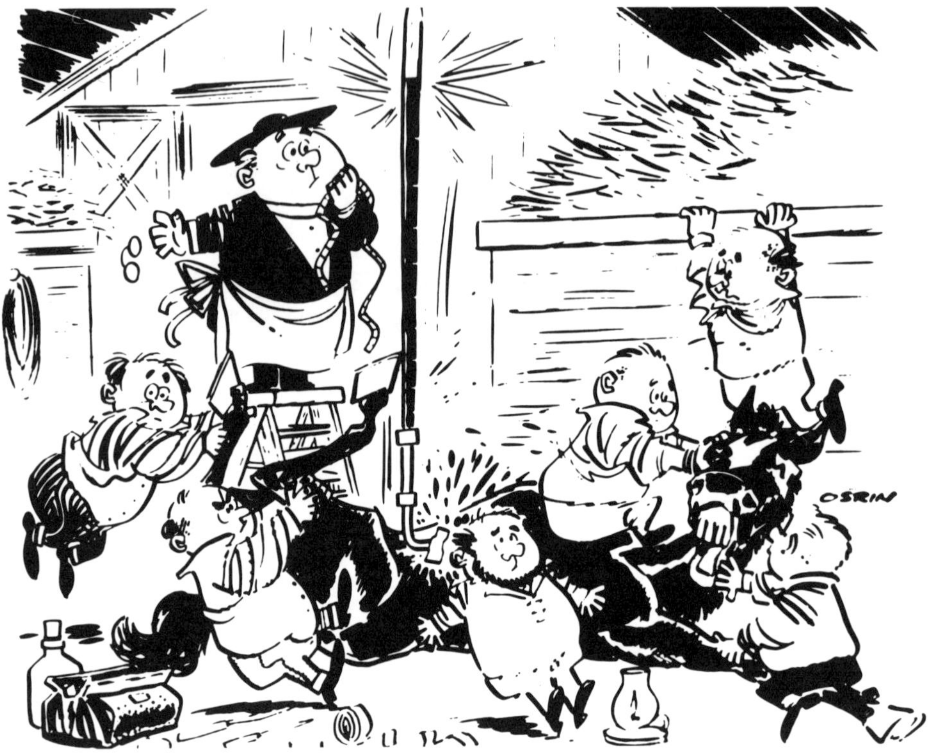

Artist's conception of the scene in the laboratory (barn) of the Reverend Stephen Hales when he first noted, in 1711 or 1726, but reported in his article in 1733, the interarterial blood pressure of a horse. Hales' description follows: "I caused a mare to be tied down on her back—having laid open the left crural artery, I inserted into it a brass pipe—and fixed a glass tube—nine feet in length—the blood rose in the tube eight feet three inches [calculated as 183 mm Hg] above the left ventricle of the heart—it rushed up about halfway in an instant and afterwards gradually with each pulse—the pulse of a horse that is well, and not terrified or in pain, is about 36 beats in a minute—this mare's pulse beat about 55 times in a minute and sometimes 60 or 100 she being in pain." Thus, it would appear that the Reverend Hales described the pressor response to a noxious stimulus at the same time he first observed the hydraulic force of the circulating blood.

Hypertension and Stress
A Unified Concept

Alvin P. Shapiro, MD
Shadyside Hospital, Pittsburgh, PA
and
Professor Emeritus of Medicine
University of Pittsburgh School of Medicine

LAWRENCE ERLBAUM ASSOCIATES, PUBLISHERS
1996 Mahwah, New Jersey

Lawrence Erlbaum Associates, Inc., Publishers
10 Industrial Avenue
Mahwah, New Jersey 07430

Library of Congress Cataloging-in-Publication Data

Shapiro, Alvin P. (Alvin Philip), 1920–
Hypertension and stress : a unified concept / Alvin P. Shapiro.
p. cm.
Includes bibliographical references and index.
ISBN 0-8058-1904-5 (c : alk. paper)
1. Hypertension—Psychosomatic aspects. 2. Stress (Psychology) 3. Stress (Physiology) I. Title. III. Series.
RC685.H8S497 1996
616.1'32—dc20 95-52714
CIP

Books published by Lawrence Erlbaum Associates are printed on acid-free paper, and their bindings are chosen for strength and durability.

Printed in the United States of America
10 9 8 7 6 5 4 3 2 1

Contents

Preface

I have written this book to explain the apparent dichotomy displayed by my seemingly discordant and diverse interests in hypertensive disease over the past 50 years. I have made physiological and pharmacological contributions to the understanding of hypertension and have been an active clinician in treating many patients with hypertension both as their primary internist as well as a consultant. As such, I have been a participant with colleagues of similar interests in the development of knowledge of this disorder over the years. Yet, during all of this time, I have had a major concern about the role of psychological and behavioral events on the course of hypertension, which rose out of the fact that my background had included training in psychiatry and psychosomatic disease. This latter interest has caused my fellow internists and clinical investigators to refer to me as a behaviorist/psychiatrist, whereas my colleagues in psychosomatic and behavioral science consider me to be one who contributes knowledge of cardiovascular physiology and clinical pharmacology in their midst.

I have tried to explain to both groups that there is no dichotomy in my thinking about the different aspects of this disease, and at times I have been successful in persuading some of my students of this fact. Stress factors in hypertension are as real as biochemical sequences and indeed are transmitted by the same metabolic pathways, and, accordingly, a unified concept of stress and hypertension is possible and necessary. I attempt to present such a thesis in this volume.

ACKNOWLEDGMENTS

This book is dedicated to my wife Ruth T. and to my children, Debra and David, whose indulgence and tolerance have allowed me the time to perform the work it represents.

Over the years, many colleagues have contributed to my studies. My faculty associates, Robert H. McDonald, Joseph D. Sapira, and the late Robert E. Miller made major impacts on my concepts, and my successive departmental chiefs, the late Eugene B. Ferris, Donald Seldin, and Jack Myers provided support and encouragement. The late I. Arthur Mirsky was for many years my intellectual guru. Above all, however, I owe thanks to the now several generations of medical students and residents at the Southwestern Medical School of the University of Texas, the University of Pittsburgh, and the Presbyterian-University and Shadyside Hospitals in Pittsburgh, who provided the spark, along with my patients, to ignite the research I have done. And the flame so ignited has been fanned and nurtured by a group of devoted fellows over the years. These include: Francis L. Drew, Roger Jones, John Misage, Richard Gaskill, Speros Moutsos, Eileen T. Scheib, Robert Pilewski, Richard Moriarty, James Nicotero, G. G. Geyskes, Virginia Beamer, Franz H. Leenen, Henri Turrian, Yehuda Traub, Eliseo Perez-Stabile, Daniel Redmond, Herbert Kahn, Emanuel Krifcher, Richard Reeves, Richard Lipman, Clinton Corder, A. Margareta Johnsen, Gail Rutan, Matthew Muldoon, J. Kimberly Karschner.

Finally, I am indebted to the secretarial assistance recently and over the years of Judy Maringo, Ruth Hines, Linda Marts, and Lisa Gregorius, while Melinda Fetkovich and, again, my wife Ruth T., generously have contributed their library skills.

—Alvin P. Shapiro

1

Historical Considerations

Arterial hypertension, high blood pressure (BP), has been described as a clinical entity only since the early 20th century when the works of Riva-Rocci[1] in 1896 and Korotkoff in 1905[2] led to a simple, noninvasive method of measuring BP in man. Actually, the knowledge that the circulating blood exerts an hydraulic force goes back to the observations by the Reverend Stephen Hales in 1733. Hales, in a classic paper,[3] described inserting a brass pipe into the femoral artery of a mare, then connecting it to a vertical glass tube and noting that "the blood rose eight feet and three inches (i.e., 183 mm Hg) above the left ventricle of the heart." Moreover, although the relationship of the kidney to vascular disease originated from the writings of Bright on nephritis in the early 19th century,[4] it was not until 1896 that Albutt suggested the existence of an "anterenal" form of hypertension.[5] By 1920, the differentiation of primary, or essential, hypertension from that associated with glomerulonephritis had been established. In the 1930s and 1940s the renal hemodynamic changes in hypertension were clarified indicating that the kidney developed secondary functional and pathologic changes from hypertension as well as being involved de novo in the origin of certain forms of hypertensive disease.[6,7]

Nevertheless, little change occurred in the concepts of the significance of an elevated BP and its management during this period. Hypertension was diagnostically and prognostically divided into benign and malignant types; the former was typified by minimal target organ impairment and generally was well tolerated, the latter by severe renal and ophthalmologic changes (i.e., rapidly progressive renal failure and fundal hemorrhages, exudates and papilledema). Many believed that primary hypertension of the "benign" type was indeed "essential" to maintain blood flow through aging arteries and hence in fact the origin of its name. Specific therapies for hypertension did not exist, either for the forms secondary to nephritis nor for the malignant phase of the disease and certainly not for the so-called benign essential type.

This state of affairs in the therapy of hypertension is impressively illustrated in the medical history of Franklin D. Roosevelt, U.S. President from 1932 until his untimely death in 1945 at age 63 from a massive cerebral hemorrhage. That Roosevelt had crippling poliomyelitis was well known, but less attention was given to the fact that he had progressively more severe hypertension throughout his 14 years in office. His course was "benign" during most of this time, but in 1944 he developed congestive heart failure, by now recognized as a complication of his hypertension, and was treated with digitalis and mercurial diuretics, then the "state of the art" for heart failure. However, his BP remained markedly elevated and led to his central nervous system (CNS) catastrophe a year later, as the terminal complication of his hypertension. Although Roosevelt was perhaps the "most important person" in this country, and perhaps the world, at this time, and had available to him the "best of medical care," no specific therapy for hypertension per se was given to him, for the simple reason that no therapeutic agents to safely lower BP were then available[8] (Fig. 1.1).

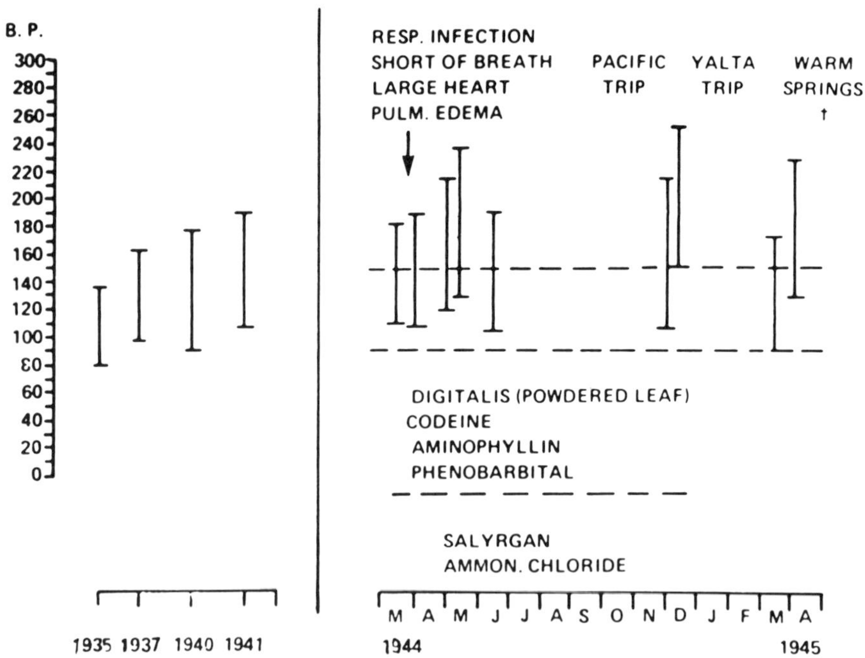

FIG. 1.1 Course of blood pressure in Franklin D. Roosevelt from 1935 to 1945 as extracted from an article by Bruenn, H. G. *Annals of Internal Medicine* (1970; 72:579–591).

I became interested in hypertension while at the Department of Medicine at the University of Cincinnati in 1948, where I completed my training in internal medicine as a fellow with Dr. Eugene B. Ferris. Dr. Ferris' research interests were broadly in the field of autonomic nervous system (ANS) control and this led to studies concerned with the sympathetic nervous system in hypertension. There were few formal training programs in the various subspecialties in medicine at that time; I suppose in modern day parlance I would be considered a fellow in general medicine. I had come back to New York City in 1947 after military service; prior to the military, I had several years of training in internal medicine, and on my return to New York City I spent approximately 9 months as a resident in psychiatry with Dr. Howard Potter of the Long Island College of Medicine and the Kings County Hospital in Brooklyn. This latter experience led to my interest in combining internal medicine and psychiatry in what was then the emerging area of psychosomatic medicine, a discipline that Dr. Ferris and others in the Departments of Medicine and Psychiatry at the University of Cincinnati were developing. As a model for psychosomatic research, they used hypertension, in which the effects of stress on the vascular system were of particular interest.

Actually, my interest in hypertension probably went back further to medical school in the early 1940s when a close relative who had hypertension also had nephrolithiasis affecting one kidney. At that time, Goldblatt's work on producing hypertension by renal arterial constriction was just beginning to attract clinical attention.[7] Actually, Tigerstedt and Bergman[9] discovered renin as a pressor agent arising from the kidney in 1897, but it was in the 1930s that Goldblatt performed his experiments in the dog in which he showed that the *ischemic* kidney could cause hypertension. It took at least 20 years after Goldblatt to work out the renin–angiotensin cycle and its relationship to ischemia, and not to parenchymal disease, of the kidney. Meanwhile, clinicians were intrigued by the possibility of "curing" hypertension by removal of a unilaterally diseased kidney of any type; hence the interest in a unilateral nephrectomy in my aforementioned relative. Fortunately, a more astute and thoughtful internist countered the enthusiasm of the urologist, and the relative had a simple nephrolithotomy, but kept his kidney and his mild hypertension, without further progression for many years.

I stayed in Cincinnati for 3 years, working primarily on mechanisms of BP control, using ganglionic blocking agents that had just been developed, as the tools for these studies. The effect of stress on BP, particularly in regard to perpetuation and progression of the disease, was also a prominent part of our work. Toward the end of this training, we did undertake early drug studies helping to develop some principles of clinical pharmacology, and more is discussed about these experiences later. Mostly our work was not in therapeutics per se. We were not further advanced from the status of therapy as described in my earlier comments about the management of Roosevelt's hypertension.

These comments thus lead to the reasons I am writing this book and constructing it in a manner related to the research in hypertension since the 1940s and 1950s. When I began to study hypertension in Cincinnati in 1948 some mechanisms were understood but the renin–angiotensin system was a speculative concept, the role of the various adrenal hormones was not known, and therapy aimed at any specific mechanism was not available. Perhaps the exception was the procedure of sympathectomy that was popular for severe hypertensives in the 1940s and was based on partial knowledge of the role of the sympathetic nervous system in hypertension. Results of this procedure were disappointing, although part of our work in Cincinnati was to develop techniques to predict who might be more amenable to this drastic surgery (i.e., by determining the acute effects of sympatholysis by ganglionic blocking agents on BP). However, the operation was largely abandoned by the 1950s.

Since the 1940s and 1950s, progress in understanding and treating hypertension has been remarkable. Although perhaps not as dramatic as the "antibiotic breakthrough" in infectious disease, this progress nevertheless has made a major contribution to health care as concerns quality of life, prevention of disability, and mortality. Hypertension and hypertensive disease had been a "silent scourge" when I first became involved in 1948, but in 1996, it is an industry. Research has expanded into the fields of epidemiology, endocrinology, surgery, pharmacology, behavioral medicine, and others. Therapeutic accomplishments have made hypertension a leading source of income for the pharmaceutical industry and the field of clinical pharmacology really originated with the development of drugs used to treat hypertension. Increasingly, specific drugs to treat specific mechanisms that raise BP have come from the laboratory to the bedside. Many physicians of various specialties treat hypertension today; it is a disorder commonly and frequently treated in the outpatient practices of family practitioners, general internists, cardiologists, and even many of the other subspecialties within internal medicine.

Throughout all these developments, a constant awareness has been present that emotional stress, both from within the individual as well as from environmental sources, plays a role in the predisposition, precipitation, and perpetuation of hypertension. Arguments have been put forth that such stress may be the major cause of at least some forms of hypertension, to the thesis that although some effect is present from stress, it is only a minor perturbation of no significance in the overall pattern of the disease. Advocates of stress theory may be biased by a lack of detailed knowledge or experience with the physiology and biochemistry involved in the establishment of this disorder but on the other hand, those who deny the importance of stress factors may be unaware of the large body of data that indicate the role of these factors in any comprehensive understanding of hypertension.

Our own approach to hypertension follows from the Mosaic Theory, which the late Irving Page brilliantly advocated for many years.[10] In this concept, multiple factors can be invoked in understanding the etiology and management of hypertension, with the strength of the individual factors varying depending on genetic background, acquired diseases, and environmental influences. Stress can be involved in predisposition by affecting a genetically programmed person, in precipitation by supplying the stimulus to bring the disease to a clinical level, and in perpetuation by maintaining or exacerbating the clinical disease. Accordingly, in this book I attempt to integrate what is known about the effects of stress on BP with the overall mosaic of the disease, hypertension, so as to underline where, in Page's

Mosaic, these factors are best fitted. In this effort, I make use of the aforementioned "three Ps"—predisposition, precipitation, and perpetuation—as part of the framework for this integration, a concept developed by the late I. Arthur Mirsky as a device by which to study behavioral impacts in psychosomatic disease.[11]

REFERENCES

1. Riva-Rocci S. Un novo sfigmanometro. *Gazz Med Torino.* 1896;47:981–1017.
2. Korotkoff NS. On methods of studying blood pressure. *Izvestiya Voenno-Med Akad.* 1905;11:365–367.
3. Hales S. *Statical essays: Containing hemostatics; An account of some hydraulik and hydrostatical experiments.* 2nd ed., London: Innys and Mandy; 1740: 1–3.
4. Bright R. Tabular view of the morbid appearances in 100 cases connected with albuminous urine with observations. *Guy's Hosp Rep.* 1836;1:380.
5. Albutt TC. Senile plethora or high arterial pressure in elderly persons. *Trans Hunter Soc.* 1895;77:38.
6. Goldring W, Chasis H, Ranges HA, Smith HW. Effective renal blood flow in patients with essential hypertension. *J Clin Invest.* 1941;20:637.
7. Goldblatt H, Lynch J, Hanzal RF, Summerville NW. Studies on experimental hypertension. I. The production of persistent elevation of systolic blood pressure by means of renal ischemia. *J Exp Med.* 1934;59:347.
8. Bruenn HG. Clinical notes on the illness and death of President Franklin D. Roosevelt. *Ann Intern Med.* 1970;72:579–591.
9. Tigerstedt R, Bergman PG. Niere und Krieslauf. *Skand Arch Physiol.* 1898;8:223.
10. Page IH. The nature of arterial hypertension. *Arch Intern Med.* 1963;111:103–115.
11. Mirsky IA. Physiologic, psychologic and social determinants in the etiology of duodenal ulcer. *Am J Dig Dis.* 1958;3:285–314.

2

Reactivity and Blood Pressure

ACUTE BLOOD PRESSURE REACTIVITY

The most obvious reason for implicating stress as a factor in hypertension is the observation of the lability of BP which occurs with almost any perturbation of the organism. *Reactivity* has been defined as the individual's propensity to display BP changes when encountering stimuli that are engaging, challenging, or aversive. Such stimuli may arise from the environment or from within the individual, and may be pleasant as well as noxious.

Reactivity should be differentiated from variability. Variability is the tendency for BP to vary on repeated measurement over time—minute to minute, daily, weekly, and so on; it is a biological phenomenon with many causes, whereas reactivity is the response of the BP to stimuli. Reactivity can be depressor as well as pressor; in fact, as is discussed later, the reduction of BP that occurs with certain behavioral manipulations and therapies is an example of the converse of the pressor response to stimuli, which is then a depressor response.

Reactivity has been measured in the laboratory by a wide variety of stimuli, both physical and psychological. The former include the cold pressor (CP) test, ischemic pain, intravenous injections—ranging from saline (placebo) to various catecholamines—exercise, smoking, hypercarbia, hyperventilation, and so forth. Psychological stimuli that have been popular in various studies include mental arithmetic in various forms, mirror tracing, the Stroop Color–Word test, role-playing by the investigators, interviews concerning known stressful topics, video games, speech tasks, and introduction of coping problems.[1] The reactivity response is usually measured as the arithmetic difference between the baseline BP and the estimated peak of the stress reaction, but in some studies a baseline adjustment is considered by using a percentile response. Manuck, in his recent writings considered that such a baseline adjustment allows a better measure of actual reactivity as contrasted with variability.[2]

Many problems are associated with the interpretation of reactivity as it is seen in the laboratory; Manuck has recently reviewed these extensively.[2] One of the obvious concerns is the relationship of laboratory responses to the reactivity and variability seen in "real life" and the evidence for correlations between these two measurements is quite mixed. Although such correlations have been considered and debated for several decades, the relatively recent availability of reliable ambulatory monitors has permitted inroads to be made on this question. Present status is summarized in a comprehensive review by Turner et al.[3] who concluded "on the basis of all the empirical evidence—there is moderate evidence for an association between laboratory and field cardiovascular activity." These authors based their conclusion on a review of 32 studies that examined laboratory reactivity as compared to specific field stressors, and to self-monitored BPs or ambulatory BP assessments in the field. The strongest correlations, at the .6 to .7 level, were seen between laboratory and field mean levels of cardiovascular activity, but were inconsistent in regard to laboratory and field reactivity, and between laboratory reactivity and field levels. (It is unclear, but the authors seem to use the terms *cardiovascular activity* and *cardiovascular reactivity* interchangeably.)

It seems somewhat optimistic to use these admittedly inconsistent results to argue that convincing evidence exists for an association of laboratory and field reactivity, or that variability seen in real-life situations can be reliably predicted. Light et al. published a study[4] in which levels of BP in a select cohort showed some relationship to reactivity measures determined over a decade earlier to a coping task, but it is a retrospective observation not originally designed for the purpose for which it was used. One observation of interest that emerges from the Turner et al.[3] review is that reactivity to psychological stressors in the lab is more closely related to field variability than reactivity to physical stressors. The authors also appropriately pointed out that other influences in the environment such as physical activity, posture, diurnal variation, and various bodily functions (e.g., fullness of the bladder) affect variability in an unpredictable fashion. Added to these, various illnesses such as diabetes mellitus, which affect the ANS, as well as age, temperature, and medications will further influence variability.

The "real-world" considerations also include many other confounding factors that modulate reactivity. Genetic patterns, acquired disease (particularly of the kidney), sodium and body fluid status, and ethnic and racial origins all will affect reactivity, whereas intrapersonal tensions, interpersonal relationships, occupational stresses, coping problems, and social support are among the influences on BP levels and the degree of variability displayed by the individual. The majority of these factors have been subjected to studies over the years, and yield tempting but similarly inconsistent data toward resolving the problem of how stress fits into the overall pattern of hypertensive disease.

In regard to the BP changes, a great deal of attention has been paid to elucidating and understanding the hemodynamics of reactivity and variability. Investigators have looked at systolic (SBP) and diastolic blood pressure (DBP), alone and separately; mean BP, both direct and calculated; and heart rate (HR); and tried to make meaningful interpretations of what these mean, individually and collectively, in regard to whether responses are perturbations of cardiac output or peripheral resistance. Cardiac output is a function of stroke volume and HR and an increase generally is evidenced in rises in SBP. Peripheral resistance, and DBP, may actually decline with some stimuli, such as aerobic exercise, which cause an increase in cardiac output. Other stimuli, such as the CP and ischemic pain, seem to cause primarily a diastolic elevation, often with no change or even a drop in HR. In earlier studies therefore, assumptions about whether BP change was largely due to cardiac output or peripheral resistance change were made on the basis of the relative degree of systolic or diastolic pressor response and over the years, both reactivity and the stimuli have been classified into "cardiac versus vascular" reactors and stimulators.[1,2] Because established hypertension is generally thought to be a disease of increased peripheral resistance, more attention has been given to those reactions that are primarily diastolic in regards to evaluating their potential impact on predicting, precipitating, and potentiating hypertension.

In recent years, however, this simple paradigm has lost some of its specificity and significance, for several reasons. First of all, systolic levels of BP have increasingly been shown to have prognostic value at least equal to that of diastolic levels, particularly in older persons, whereas in younger individuals systolic reactivity may be prominent and may switch to diastolic reactivity in a later stage of the disorder. Second, although the type of response may vary among different stimuli, a given stimulus may also vary in the type of response it elicits. In addition, medications and probably other conditions as well, such as sympathetic nervous system afflictions, can affect the type of response.

In the 1950s and 1960s, we reported a group of studies of reactivity to a number of simple stimuli. The stimuli included a 10 ml. injection of normal saline accompanied by the requirement of the patient to count to 100, a repeat of this test with the patient being required to count backward as rapidly as possible (Saline and Saline-R), a CP test with the hand immersed in cold water for 1 minute, and a Stroop test (Color). The Saline tests and the Color test were considered as "emotional stimuli" and produced responses that were predominantly systolic with a systolic/diastolic ratio of greater than 2.0; the CP test was considered a "physical stimulus" affecting peripheral resistance and was predominately diastolic with an S/D ratio of 1.4. The diastolic response to the CP test was significantly greater than that to the Saline and Color tests, but within the group there were some individuals who displayed a prominent diastolic response to these "emotional stimuli" (Fig. 2.1). This was most evident in younger males, whereas older individuals had more prominent systolic responses.[5] In present day nomenclature, these responses would be considered as contrasting vascular reactors (peripheral resistance responses) to cardiac reactors (cardiac output responses) but of course such hemodynamic measurements by direct means were not available at that time.

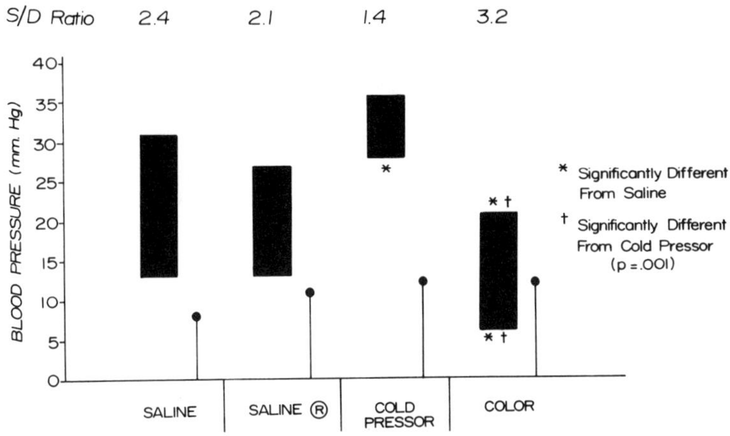

FIG. 2.1. Average response to four different noxious stimuli in 50 hypertensive patients. the upper border of each black bar represents the systolic pressure; the lower edge is the diastolic. The vertical lines with the black circles indicate the average pulse rate.

This group of hypertensives included a number of patients receiving antihypertensive drugs, primarily sympatholytics and thiazides. It was noted that the responses of these treated patients were not significantly less than those of the untreated patients. In several subsequent studies, this observation was tested in a controlled manner. Patients treated with reserpine and chlorothiazide, separately and combined, were noted to have responses that were not significantly different before and during treatment, although the "ceiling pressures" achieved were lower during treatment because the basal pressures had of course been lowered. Also noted was a change in the pattern of the response in some of the patients, particularly those on reserpine, who had an increased diastolic response; this was interpreted as possibly indicating that the sympathetic denervation produced by the norepinephrine-depleting drug, reserpine, rendered their peripheral vessels "supersensitive" to any humoral mediators of the pressor response.[6] In a subsequent study, in which guanethidine sulfate and alpha methyl dopa were used in treatment, these more potent sympatholytic drugs did diminish responsiveness modestly, but in keeping with the supposition that sympatholysis might render the vessels supersensitive to humoral agents, the response to a small intravenous injection of angiotensin II, which by this time was available, was increased.[7]

Subsequently, we undertook a study of the responses to these stimuli in normotensive and hypertensive diabetics and nondiabetics and observed differences in magnitude and patterns of reactivity related to both the presence and absence of hypertension as well as to diabetes. Thus, hypertensives were more responsive to all the tests employed, including the Saline and Color tests as well as the CP test and the injection of angiotensin II. On the other hand, diabetics demonstrated reduced responses to the CP test and enhanced responses to the angiotensin II injections, presumably as a consequence of diminished sympathetic nervous system innervation, and similar to what we had previously noted in subjects receiving sympatholytic drugs. Responses to the two psychologic tests, Saline and Color, were not diminished in the diabetics, suggesting that alternate pathways to the sympathetic nervous system were available for these stimuli[8] (Figs. 2.2 and 2.3).

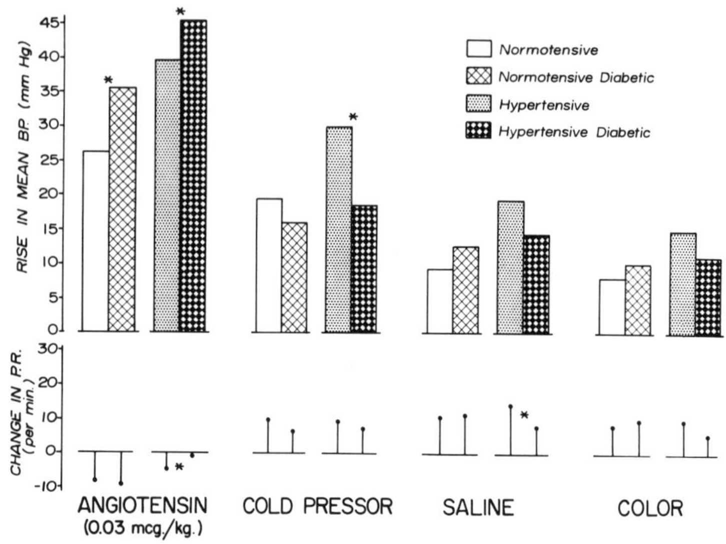

FIG. 2.2. Blood pressure and pulse rate responses to four different stimuli in the four different groups of patients indicated. The data are arranged to show the contrast between diabetic and nondiabetic groups. Significant differences ($p < .05$) are indicated by an asterisk.

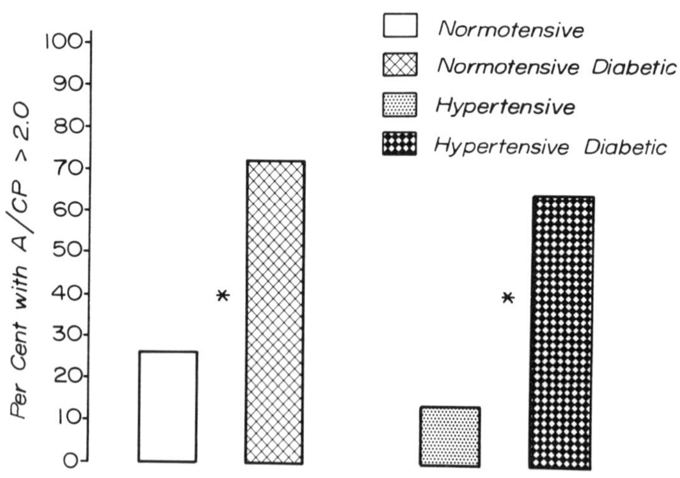

FIG. 2.3. Comparison of percentage of subjects with angiotensin/cold pressor (A/CP) ratio greater than 2.0 in the diabetic and nondiabetic groups. Significant differences ($p = < .02$ by chi-square analysis) are indicated by an asterisk.

In the course of these experiments, we also examined the responses of a group of normotensives divided into those with and without a family history of hypertension. The subjects with a positive family history displayed an increased response to the Saline, Color, and CP tests (angiotensin was not used in these studies) but it was only in the systolic component of the BP responses. This was interpreted as suggesting that although hypertension is eventually a disease of increased peripheral resistance, its earliest manifestation may be that of increased cardiac output in response to stimuli. These assumptions obviously were made without the benefit of direct measurements of cardiac output, being based on the concept, with its aforementioned flaws, that elevation of systolic BP reflected increased cardiac output whereas diastolic rises indicated peripheral resistance increase.[5]

In a later study, we examined the effect of the beta blocker, propranolol, on the response to the CP test and to ischemic pain. A diminution in the HR response was noted to these stimuli, but the BP rise was not affected. In some of the patients, actual cardiac output was determined, using a dye dilution technique, and this response was less while receiving the beta blocker, and in fact in several of the patients it actually fell, although the pressor response was maintained. Urinary catecholamine excretion consequent to the stimuli, was not decreased. These findings were interpreted as indicating that blocking the inotropic and chronotropic cardiac components of the pressor response was counteracted by the enhanced response of the alpha receptors—supersensitivity again—with enhanced vasoconstriction and increased peripheral resistance.[9] Subsequently, similar findings were observed with another beta blocker, practolol, in a group of hypertensive patients.[10]

Two other studies during this sequence of our work are worthy of note in regard to the pathways of pressor reactivity. In the first of these, we noted differences in magnitude of responses to CP testing and ischemic pain, without evidence of a relationship between these differences and adrenergic activation, as measured by catecholamine excretion and free fatty acid mobilization. In fact, the evidence suggested that change in adrenergic activation related to the order in which the stimuli were presented (e.g., higher activity when the experience was novel) rather than to the nature of the stimulus or the degree of response.[11] The second study was an analysis of responses in monozygotic (MZ) and dizygotic (DZ) twins, which revealed concordance of cardiovascular responses greater in the MZs, but discordance of the adrenergic activation, further suggesting that although genetic composition had something to do with reactivity, it was a function of the intrinsic cardiovascular mechanism of response, and not on the degree of sympathetic activation alone.[12]

In retrospect, and in light of present day emerging knowledge about the molecular factors that influence peripheral cardiac and vascular reactivity—which are discussed further in a later chapter—what we may have been observing at that time was that genetic traits guide hemodynamic responses perhaps through stimulation of endothelial mechanisms rather than the adrenergic system.

To sum up our observations from this series of studies in the laboratory, we concluded that reactivity to stimuli was a component of variability of BP but that both the magnitude and the patterns of response were in themselves quite mixed.

Thus, genetic influences, other illness, sociocultural status, medications, availability and status of neurogenic/humoral response pathways, age, gender, the interpersonal tensions of the subject and his or her perception of the environment, and of course the character and the nature of the stimulus itself, all were factors in determining the elicitation of a response, its hemodynamic pattern and its magnitude. With these considerations, it seems difficult to believe that one can predict a given response, and most importantly, predict the future development of significant clinical hypertension from the reactivity component of lability on the basis of pressor responsiveness either in the laboratory or in the field. Thus, we proposed the hypothesis that stress and hypertension relate in a quantitative fashion, rather than a qualitative one, namely that the sum total of reactive experience over time is the determining influence on the development of disease and not the precise pattern of the response or even the individual's substrate. With this analysis one can account for two of the three Ps, perpetuation and perhaps precipitation, albeit not for predictability.

It would seem also that these observations are in keeping with the hypothesis propounded by Julius of the hemodynamic plasticity involved in pressor responsivity. Julius argued that the "CNS seeks a level of blood pressure under various stimulus conditions and will regulate the circulation to accomplish this end even when customary pressor mechanisms are not available."[13] Thus, when the pathways for increased autonomic tone are not available, other mechanisms, perhaps humoral, perhaps peripheral/molecular, will operate integrated at the CNS level to produce the pressor response. Manuck, in discussing this hypothesis, suggested that central regulation of the pressor response independent of the proximate mechanisms invoked to elevate pressure, also dictates a pressor response of varying magnitude among individuals.[2] Similarly, a given stimulus although it may primarily invoke a response that is cardiac under most circumstances, may with changes in the individual, due to age, drugs, and so on, produce a response of the same pressor magnitude that is now a vasoconstrictive increase.

Page commented about reactivity and predictability in stating that measurements of cardiovascular reactivity have "yielded an extraordinarily mixed bag of results." He pointed out for instance that the cold pressor test that was emphasized as a predictor of hypertension had fallen into disuse because of inconsistency of results and that discrepancies also appear in tests of reactivity of various special vascular beds, such as the retina and the nail bed. He concluded that the response of arterial BP is too broadly based to be of specific value in prediction and prognosis and concludes that "thirty-five years after initiation of studies of reactivity, there is still insufficient agreement either to allow dogmatic statements or to insure clinical usefulness."[14] On the other hand, several more recent reports, by Wood et al.[15] and by Menkes et al.[16] have reawakened some interest in the CP test as a predictor of future risk of hypertension. The report by Wood et al. comprised a follow-up of subjects for up to 45 years whereas that of Menkes et al. looked at a follow-up for 20 to 36 years. One might hope that further long-term studies such as these two might serve to counter Page's skepticism, but personally I am inclined to agree with his doubts both because of the difficulty of maintaining a well controlled study for a long period of time as well as for the fact that, as he clearly stated, the BP responses are so multiply determined that a laboratory response to a single test can be quite misleading.

These considerations may leave reactivity per se only as a fascinating epiphenomenon in the etiology and development of hypertension in general and essential hypertension in particular. It is observed at all times and affects decisions as to prognosis and management and may well influence the course of the disease, but it is not causal except in its quantitative impact over time as an additive to the basal BP state of the individual. In other words, there must be "something there" to begin with; the reactivity (and variability) serve to produce the lability that we observe clinically, but does not necessarily predict the disease or produce it.

STRESS AND CHRONIC HYPERTENSION IN HUMANS

I have discussed the concept of *reactivity* as the mechanism by which stress transduces hypertension acutely and thereby chronically. However, there are other reasons why stress has been implicated in a causal relationship to the disease. These reasons include the retrospective correlations between emotional events, both personal and environmental, and the apparent precipitation, perpetuation, and aggravation of hypertensive disease.

Historically, insights into relationships between behavior and somatic disease are first derived from attempts to correlate the time when a disease started or became aggravated with temporally related behavioral events. Thus, a cardiovascular disorder beginning at some given point and associated with a change in the environment or personal behavior of the patient that elicited an emotional stress permits an assumption that the stress was concerned with the production of the disease.

In this manner observers such as Wolf,[17] Binger,[18] Reiser,[19] and their coworkers provided data indicating the relationships between certain emotional trauma in the past history of individuals and the onset or acceleration of hypertensive disease and other cardiovascular ailments.

An example of this approach is the study by Reiser et al. of 230 patients with varying types and severity of hypertension. They focused on the natural history of the disease in the individual patients, the time relationships of emotionally stressful life situations to the previous course and symptoms of the illness, and the psychodynamic meaning of the life-situation change to the particular patient. Thus, they examined not only whether a change occurred but whether a seemingly innocuous emotional event was nevertheless of significant meaning in terms of the particular psychodynamic background of the individual.

With this technique, whereas correlations between emotional events and physical manifestations of hypertensive illness were noted in only 9% of those patients who were seen for medical survey only, the correlations rose to 63% in those who were studied psychiatrically as well as medically during initial diagnostic contact.

In those patients in whom sustained relationships developed, the incidence of correlations rose from approximately 50% in those who were followed primarily medically, to 100% in the patients who were followed medically and psychiatrically. In other words, the more intensively the investigators looked at life situations and their impact, the more frequently correlations were found. Moreover, repetitiveness of an emotional trauma that had specific meaning to the patient was noted to correlate highly with exacerbation and even acceleration of the hypertension from the benign to the malignant phase.[20,19]

Similar data are available from papers by Weiss et al.,[21] Fischer,[22] Hambling,[23] Van der Valk,[24] and others reviewed by Weiner.[25] However, these data suffer from the obvious defect of all retrospective analyses. The correlations may be simply coincidental or biased while the prevalence of similar events in people who do not develop hypertension is not controlled. Koch's postulates cannot be fulfilled because it is difficult to isolate the "pathogen" and impossible, if it were isolated and identified, to reintroduce it into a similar host. Nevertheless, it is of interest that the research on life-change events by Holmes and Rahe[26] have suggested correlations between precipitation of many diseases and the sum total of ordinary life events. What continues to be an enigma is whether the type of disease resulting from life stress is a consequence of stimulus specificity, the quantitative "total" of the stress, or the "nature of the substrate" (i.e., the predisposed organ systems of the host).

A retrospective study that is really prospective, and does have "controls," is that reported by Timio et al. in 1988.[27] This group of investigators examined the BP in a group of 144 nuns in a secluded and cloistered order, over a period of 20 years, and compared them with a group of 138 laywomen living in the areas surrounding the nunnery in Umbria, Italy. BPs determined every 4 years in the two groups showed a striking discrepancy; in the laywomen the pressures gradually rose, whereas in the nuns BPs remained essentially the same. At the end of 20 years, the average BP in the laywomen was approximately 162/90 mm Hg, whereas in the nuns it was 120/80 mm Hg. The investigators examined various aspects of lifestyle other than the obvious difference between women living in an interactive society and those living the cloistered, protected lives of the nuns. They found no differences in salt intake, body mass index, menarche and menopause, family history, or the use of stimulants between the two groups. Nor did childbirth provide a difference in BP among the laywomen and consequently could not have played a role in the higher pressures of the laywomen as a group. Moreover, there was a somewhat paradoxical finding in the fact that cholesterol and triglyceride levels were actually higher in the nuns, which the investigators attributed to the "generally lipid-rich diet with low physical activity in the nunneries."

These rather impressive findings suggesting that a "simple" lifestyle seems to confer protection against the development of hypertension are in keeping with a number of older studies in unacculturated societies in which BP has been noted to remain normal with aging; these include studies in the Solomons, in Fiji, New Guinea, and Brazil, in some of which pressure may actually fall with age.[28,29,30] In the primitive societies, which—although "simple" in terms of what we consider the stresses of modern day culture—can scarcely be called unstressful in terms of survival, the failure of BP to rise and to actually fall has been interpreted by some as a nutritional deficit, but this cannot be considered a factor in the well-fed, even cholesterolemic, nuns. What then are the circumstances in lifestyle that differ among the nuns in contrast to the laywomen in the same area? Timio et al. pointed out that the main differences are less anxiety for their earthly future; less drive, competition, and expectations; less economic and familial stress; less social and political tensions; and decreased exposure to noise and pollution. The authors concluded that living in this low stress environment with freedom from most sources of human conflict over the 20 years of the observational period prevented the development of hypertension among them, albeit by mechanisms unknown.[27]

Although not directly connected with hypertension or its development, the findings in this group of nuns resemble the observations of Bruhn and Wolf in the population of Rosetto, Pennsylvania in which a closely knit group of Italian immigrants were noted to have a significantly lower incidence of morbidity and mortality from cardiovascular disease than their neighbors in surrounding communities despite lack of dietary control of lipids. Wolf attributed their protection against heart disease to the close and paternalistic nature of the society that kept them immune from outside community pressures.[31] In a sense, this society was "cloistered and secluded" like the nunnery. Indeed, as Wolf and Bruhn pointed out recently, the inroads of modern society on the Rosetto community have resulted in a breakdown of its close ties and family dominance and has in turn been associated with a disappearance of the lower incidence of heart disease.[32]

As a counterpoint to these group instances of "protection" from hypertension, are examples of hypertension developing in populations following major catastrophic events. These include the often quoted observation by Ruskin et al.[33] of hypertension developing in survivors of the Texas City disaster, an oil tanker explosion in its harbor that leveled a good part of the city. Graham described development of transient hypertension after desert combat in World War II[34] and similarly, Miasnikov[35] commented on an increased prevalence of hypertension developing in Leningrad following its lengthy siege in World War II. And yet, despite intense stress that existed in populations throughout this period—populations exposed to mass bombings, acts of terrorism, imprisonment and threats of extermination—the three reports listed here seem to be all that are recorded, leading one to wonder that perhaps they are isolated observations with inadequate control groups that can only be considered on an anecdotal level. On the other hand, aside from these major catastrophic events, strong evidence for the effect of environmental and behavioral stimuli have come from epidemiologic investigations that have shown a relationship between elevated BP and a number of environmental variables that presumably have in common their stressful content. These data have been reviewed by Henry and Stephens[36] and by Gutman and Benson[37] who point out that urban populations tend to have higher BPs and that standard of living, income, education, and type of occupation are associated with differences in BP levels. Data are available,[38] albeit inconsistent and not confirmed by others,[39] that the coefficient of resemblance of BP levels is greater not only in blood-related family members but also between spouses, suggesting environmental and cultural as well as genetic influences.

It seems clearly established that the Black population of the United States has a higher prevalence of elevated BP than do Whites. Less certain are implications that the difference is greater in "high-stress" neighborhoods and has a relationship to socioeconomic status (SES); more educated or high-income Blacks have less hypertension,[40] but in Mississippi, rural women have higher BP than do urban women.[41] Elevated BP has also been associated with rapid cultural change in several areas of the world and with socioeconomic mobility.[36] A potent argument can be developed, although ingenuous and easily refuted, that contemporary people are faced with the continuous stress of conflict and uncertainty that leads to cardiovascular adjustments appropriate to physical actions taken in a primitive society but that can no longer be utilized and resolved in present day civilized society.

In summary, epidemiologic studies, although a rich source of provocative data, provide only limited understanding of the pathogenesis of hypertension as related to stress, since they fail to account for the selectivity of the sociocultural impact on the development of hypertension in a given population. Moreover, they are not experiments that can be readily reversed by removing the supposed pathogen, and they are retrospective. Yet, they emphasize the need to study the influences of both group and individual behavior, in conjunction with genetic susceptibility, diet, sodium intake, and the other physiologic factors, in evaluating the prevalence of hypertension in different populations. Again, the impact of stress may be quantitative, or massive, rather than qualitative.

STUDIES OF STRESS AND HYPERTENSION IN ANIMALS

Many attempts to produce hypertension by long-term exposure of rats to stress have been reported. Early studies used audiogenic stimuli and were able to produce hypertension that lasted as long as the stimulus was continued.[42] Repeated electric shock has not been effective in producing chronic hypertension in rats,[43] although there is evidence that steroids, renin activity, and pressor response to angiotensin will increase with such procedures.[44,45,46] Electric shock in rats with a predisposition to hypertension from several different kinds of renal injury has produced chronic BP elevations earlier or beyond that seen in control animals.[47,48] These studies are reviewed further (v.i.).

A series of studies by Dahl and coworkers in their strain of salt-sensitive rats (i.e., rats that develop hypertension when exposed to a high salt intake, in contrast to their controls) failed to show chronic elevation of BP when an aversive Pavlovian conditioning procedure was used (i.e., electric shock administered independent of the rat's behavior).[49] However, Friedman and Dahl then studied the salt-sensitive strain using a long-term aversive conflict situation and were able to produce significant elevation of BP.[50,51] Folkow has noted that spontaneously hypertensive rats (SHR) during their prehypertensive state are more responsive than controls to noxious stimuli, showing increased beta-adrenergic activity.[52]

A number of studies have been done in monkeys using avoidance conditioning. Studies by Benson, Herd, and collaborators[53] and Forsythe[54] produced long-term elevations of BP in monkeys that have been associated occasionally with some cardiac pathology.

One of the more striking demonstrations is the series of experiments reported by Henry et al.[55,56] in mice. These investigators produced sustained elevations in SBP in mouse colonies consequent to exposure to the psychosocial stimulus of "crowding" the living space of the animals and forcing them to compete for territory. Their studies are unique and imaginative because they reproduce in an animal model the type of psychosocial condition that has been proposed as significant in the epidemiologic correlations noted in humans. Henry et al. also looked at pathologic changes in kidney and heart occurring with the hypertension, as well as mechanisms, particularly those concerned with the ANS and norepinephrine metabolism. Recently, Henry et al. have also described production of mild hypertension in rats using their psychosocial stress model. It is noteworthy that these outcomes differed markedly depending on the strain of rat that they studied.[57]

Our own experiments in regard to production of hypertension in animals began in 1955 with studies of cats who were subjected to a procedure designed to produce experimental neurosis and anxiety. We used the paradigm described by Masserman that entailed the introduction of a food–shock conflict and measured BP by direct arterial puncture repeatedly over a period averaging almost 1 year. Although it was noted that the basal BPs of these felines were somewhat high and that occasional further elevations were noted during the repeated readings, no sustained elevations were achieved and control animals—not subjected to the conditioning procedure—did not differ significantly in their BPs than the experimental animals. Several of the cats were subjected to an ischemic kidney injury—figure-of-eight tie of one kidney*—and showed a slight increase in basal BP, but no further rise with conditioning. Pathological examination of the kidneys and hearts of a number of the animals failed to show any vascular lesions of hypertension. Of interest also in this study were measures of serum pepsinogen, at that time thought to be a possible marker of a tendency to peptic ulcer. No significant changes in pepsinogen levels were noted but there was a quite significant *inverse* correlation between levels of BP and levels of pepsinogen (i.e., cats with higher pepsinogen had lower BPs and vice versa). Behavioral changes in the cats were not apparent so that although we concluded that the Masserman experimental neurosis would not produce lasting hypertensive disease in the cat, even after modest renal injury, the degree of psychological disturbance was considered not sufficient to rule out the possibility that other types of stress might be more productive. We were impressed by the inverse relationship between the BP and the pepsinogen and suggested that this was in keeping with speculation current at that time about psychosomatic

*A "figure of eight tie of one kidney" is a constricting ligature around the kidney designed to produce renal ischemia.

disease specificity as it related to sympathetic and parasympathetic components of the ANS.[58]

Continuing these studies that attempted to produce hypertension in animals by a psychologically disturbing exposure, we then, in 1956, subjected rats to an avoidance conditioning experience over a period of 10 weeks. The rats were divided into a group that received a high salt intake and those on a normal intake; controls were unstressed groups with and without the increased salt intake. BP was slightly higher in the "salted" animals, reflected also in a slightly higher heart weight, but identical in the stressed and unstressed animals. The effectiveness of the psychostimulation paradigm that we employed was demonstrated by the fact that adrenal size was increased in the stressed rats. At that time, we interpreted these data to mean that this type of stress was insufficient in severity or duration to produce hypertension and/or that the high salt intake was an inadequate targeting for producing or exacerbating hypertension with stress.[44] It is of interest that Anderson and coworkers some years later, in 1983 and again in 1987,[59,60] studied dogs exposed to avoidance conditioning while receiving saline infusions and demonstrated a rise in BP during the continuation of these procedures for several weeks. However, when the saline and stress were discontinued, the hypertension receded. Their reports do not indicate that any pathological changes of hypertension occurred in these animals. Although one may speculate that longer exposure might lead to a permanent state of hypertension, the fact remains that we still do not have a clear-cut demonstration of chronic hypertension produced by a stress paradigm. With Haythornthwaite and Pradley, Anderson recently studied a group of normotensive students on high sodium intake during periods of high and low life stress (exam period vs. summer vacation) and noted a transient slight rise in systolic BP during the high stress, high sodium period.[61]

We made another attempt to combine stress with targeting in a study in 1957 of the effect of the avoidance conditioning technique on rats subjected to figure-of-eight tie of one kidney and contralateral nephrectomy. Rats subjected to this procedure develop fairly severe hypertension, and by the end of 36 weeks in this study all surviving rats were hypertensive and all had severe renal impairment although the actual severity of the hypertension was not correlated with the degree of renal impairment. The rats were initially divided into a group that received avoidance conditioning during the course of the experiment and a group that were followed for the same period who were not stressed. Hypertension developed more rapidly in the stressed rats, appearing at an average of 14 weeks in the stressed animals and 26 weeks in the unstressed group. Hypertensive renal damage was also significantly worse in the stressed rats.[47]

In 1958, we reported the results of a large series of studies in which rats were subjected to several different kinds of stress designed to produce psychostimulation, using a variety of nonrenal targeting techniques such as induction of a hypothyroid state and injection of catecholamine enhancing drugs. We were unsuccessful in producing significant hypertension, even on a transient basis in these animals or of gastric, cardiac, or renal damage. We did again see some adrenal enlargement in stressed animals.[43]

Some years later, in 1967 during the course of a series of studies on the relationships of hypertension to pyelonephritis in rats, we did demonstrate an example of combined stress and organ targeting. We had shown that pyelonephritis alone in rats did not produce chronic hypertension, although hypertension, both acute and chronic, did increase susceptibility to pyelonephritis. In the 1979 experiment we showed that pyelonephritic rats developed elevated BP when exposed to behavioral stimulation, although the stress alone, and pyelonephritis alone, failed to cause hypertension.[48] The mechanism for this outcome is suggested by several previous studies we had reported. In an experiment in 1964, we had shown that rats with renal hypertension, produced by renal artery clip, were hyperreactive to infused angiotensin II.[62] In another study, in 1966, normal rats who were subjected to stress also demonstrated increased responsivity to infused angiotensin II.[46] Finally, in a study in 1974, we provided data that rats exposed to intermittent electric shock developed a marked rise in plasma renin activity (PRA) which began to subside within a few hours but remained somewhat elevated for up to 24 hours. The rise was blunted by beta blockade with propranolol but exaggerated by alpha blockade with phentolamine. Hypophysectomy did not inhibit the rise in renin further indicating that the effect was mediated through sympathetic arousal.[45]

Our conclusions from this series of studies were that hypertension and stress in animals were not directly related, but required the mediation of other factors that in some way targeted the cardiovascular system. Even this conclusion, however, is not consistent but has varied over the years in studies by different investigators. Lawler, for instance, noted that different types of stress in rats with borderline hypertension resulted in more severe elevations of BP[63] but in recent reports his data are less impressive, including studies in which high salt intake was used as a provoking factor.[64] A comprehensive recent report by Gelsema et al. is particularly disappointing to advocates of the reactivity hypothesis. These investigators studied borderline hypertensive rats, on normal or high salt intakes, exposed to the psychosocial stress of aggregation housing, similar to what Henry has used in his experiments.[65] No hypertension developed in any aggregation, although most of the rats showed signs of perceived stress in terms of reduced weight gain, enlarged adrenal glands, and body wounds. Cardiac hypertrophy did ensue, which the investigators interpreted as reflecting increased physical activity and/or intermittent increases in sympathetic tone. These recent findings of Gelsema et al. are reminiscent of those that we reported back in 1958 and indicate further that even after years of study, convincing evidence to clearly establish stress de novo as a major component in producing hypertension in animals, has not emerged.

Interesting prospects for the development and study of animal models of hypertension related to stress are available from the studies of Reis and colleagues, who have produced neurogenic hypertension by lesions in the nucleus tractus solitarii (NTS) in the medulla. Such lesions abolish the baroreceptor reflexes and result in labile hypertension.[66,67] He and his colleagues (Nathan et al.) also noted that classical conditioning of cats with bilateral lesions of the NTS results in a pressor response that is five times greater than that obtained in similarly conditioned controls.[68]

Perhaps the most significant insight that can be deduced from these studies in animals is that when successful in producing chronic hypertension, the following have been present:

1. The behavioral stimulus usually involves the continual need of the animal to adjust to a stressful situation that has in it elements of constant threat and uncertainty.
2. Targeting of the cardiovascular system by genetic predisposition or acquired conditions that in themselves distort cardiovascular adjustments appears to make the stimulus more toxic.

CNS AND ANS MECHANISMS IN HYPERTENSION RELATING TO STRESS AND REACTIVITY

The environmental and internal changes that constitute stress impact on the BP through the brain and the ANS by many mechanisms. The effects are also mediated by neuroendocrine and hypothalamopituatary pathways that can be affected by mood, appetite, thirst, and other behaviors. These include influences through the renin–angiotensin system, adrenal medullary and cortical secretions, vasopressin, and peripheral vasoactive peptides, both known and as yet unknown, and more recently endothelial factors and the nitric oxide system. Central effects are also modified by the arterial baroreceptors that buffer BP changes. Psychosocial influences on the baroreceptor via the CNS provide a potential mechanism. Conway et al. observed that changes in baroreceptor gain relate to the subject passing from sleep to drowsiness and then to the waking state and to mental arithmetic, an observation that may be relevant to such aspects of BP variability as the "white coat syndrome" on one hand and the placebo effect on the other.[69] Although it may be possible that stress effects utilize changes in baroreceptor sensitivity as one of the pathways by which reactivity is mediated, the contribution of impairment of these baroreceptor control mechanisms to long-term essential hypertension are not known. There are potential reasons for such impairment that include the atheromatous changes that occur in the receptor areas in the aorta and the carotid arteries with aging and likewise through reduced perfusion in the vertebrobasilar central areas occurring as a result of atheroma in the central circulation, so that the potential for such an input into essential hypertension is present. As mentioned earlier, Reis provided data to the effect that interruption of the baroreceptor afferents or their central connections can lead to increased BP lability.[66]

Central effects on sympathetic outflow and BP are mediated through complex interactions between rostral and caudal areas in the brainstem, the hypothalamus, and the intermediolateral columns of the spinal cord. Chalmers and Pilowsky recently reviewed their work and that of many others outlining progress and present understanding of these mechanisms.[70] It is not our intention in this work to analyze these extensive contributions (Chalmers and Pilowsky have 263 references in their

12-page review), but it is clear that the interaction of peripheral and central mechanisms are constantly in play in control of BP. To quote these authors:

> Indeed, in all physiological situations, the level of BP depends on the interaction of regional vascular and myocardial mechanisms with the actions of the sympathoadrenal system and a number of powerful hormonal mechanisms including the renin–angiotensin system, the regulators of fluid volume such as aldosterone, atrial naturetic peptide, vasopressin, and other vasoactive peptides such as prostaglandins and kinins. The ultimate challenge for the study of central mechanisms regulating BP will be, therefore, not only to dissect out the central neural components responsible, but to demonstrate the particular peripheral mechanisms through which they act. (pp. 676–677)

Most of the central control is vested in the ventral portions of the medulla and include pressor areas and depressor areas and are thus both excitatory and inhibitory with the NTS as the integrating center. The whole area had been known as the vasomotor center; present work has resulted in these finer distinctions. Chalmers and Pilowsky proposed that *disinhibition* may be the key to resetting the system in a hypertensive mode. Again, in earlier work, Doba and Reis demonstrated that destruction of the NTS could cause marked lability of the BP and even fulminant hypertension,[71] whereas Chalmers and Pilowsky have shown that hypertension can be produced by destruction of the caudal ventral lateral medulla (CVLM) which is an inhibitory area. These authors also showed that inactivation of inhibitory inputs into this area can result in sustained hypertension.[70]

The "bottom line" to these complex and difficult studies of CNS and ANS mechanisms is that pathways are present for transmission of stimuli from the brain to the periphery but we are dealing with a veritable jungle of intertwining, branching, feedback loops, and other obstacles in these pathways, which makes simple connections from stress to outcome rather impossible. Obviously, most of these studies are in animal models so that applicability to humans can come only from observational studies in selective disease states and from pharmacological probes with drugs that are known to affect specific receptors. That these mechanisms are heavily involved in BP and other cardiovascular activities is certainly without question. On the other hand, that their disturbance or distortion can produce primary or essential hypertension, particularly through chronic stress, remains to this observer at least, a matter of conjecture. One still has to deal with the probability that an organ (e.g., a diseased or ischemic kidney or an arterial tree affected by a genetic vulnerability) provides the basis that allows the interpersonal, intrapersonal, or environmental stress to have its impact. Another aspect of the CNS and ANS mechanisms is whether and how these centers feedback to influence behavior and create some aspects of the particular personality of the hypertensive individual, a sequence that has influenced our own thinking and research and that is discussed in some detail later.

A somewhat different and intriguing approach to the mechanisms by which the CNS may contribute to the development of essential hypertension derives from the hypothesis proposed by Dworkin, Miller, and coworkers.[72,73] These investigators have suggested that baroreceptor stimulation results in the relief of pain and anxiety and this mechanism is stimulated by elevations of BP that in turn causes baroreceptors to fire. Against a background of stress, this baroreceptor response functions as a reward mechanism and rise in BP becomes a learned mechanism. Miller and Dworkin originally proposed this hypothesis in 1977[72] and in Dworkin's studies in animals in 1979, he showed quantitative behavioral effects of baroreceptor stimulation in animals.[73] Dworkin pointed out a number of studies in which individuals can be "taught" to raise BP, as, for example, patients with spinal cord injuries who have orthostatic hypertension and again in baboons and monkeys who can raise BP when rewarded in conditioning experiments with food or shock avoidance. Dworkin also demonstrated that in rats in which BP has been raised by a vasoconstrictor stimulus, reactivity to noxious stimuli was reduced as displayed by diminished running activity to avoid these stimuli.[73,74]

In their most recent studies of this hypothesis, with Ebert, Dworkin, et al.[75] measured pain perception as well as basal BP in a group of normotensive patients. The subjects were followed and reevaluated in regard to BP 20 months later. Measurements were also made of the degree of stress experienced by these subjects. The investigators noted that the amount of pain reduction produced by baroreceptor stimulation predicted an increase in the follow-up BP and the increase was proportional to the degree of self assessed daily stress in these subjects. Thus, among the subjects reporting the greatest amount of stress, the pain inhibition effect accounted for more than 80% of the BP variance. The sequence that Dworkin proposed from these studies is that the stress can initiate pain and anxiety, which are in turn alleviated by BP rise and baroreceptor stimulation; the latter than "relieves" the discomfort and the baroreceptor response over time becomes a reward that requires a BP rise to elicit it. Dworkin interprets these results to be evidence of a novel behavioral mechanism by which events in the environment could gradually raise a sensitive individual's basal BP and contribute to the development of essential hypertension.[74,75]

An interesting addition to the clinical literature on the relationship of reduced pain perception to hypertension comes from a recently reported study by Guasti et al.[76] These investigators examined the threshold to dental pain in hypertensive and normotensive individuals and noted a significantly higher threshold and tolerance to pain in the hypertensive subjects. It was also noteworthy that the 24-hour ambulatory pressures in these individuals had an even better correlation to the pain thresholds than did the BPs taken during the actual pain stimulus.

Other related phenomena to this hypothesis are the reports that pain sensitivity is reduced in rats with spontaneous hypertension.[77-79] The possible relationship of this decreased pain sensitivity to endogenous CNS opioids is suggested by the fact that the insensitivity is lost after administration of the opiate antagonist, naloxone, even though the latter does not affect BP.[79]

Much important work remains to be done on CNS and ANS mechanisms in BP control and their roles in stress-mediated reactivity. Some suggestions as to directions and methods are offered in a later chapter.

REFERENCES

1. Turner JR. *Cardiovascular reactivity and stress: patterns of physiological response.* New York: Plenum Press; 1994.
2. Manuck SB. Cardiovascular reactivity in cardiovascular disease: Once more into the breech. *Int J Behav Med.* 1994;1:4-31.
3. Turner JR, Ward MM, Gellman MD, Johnston DW, Light KC, Van Doornen LJP. The relationship between laboratory and ambulatory cardiovascular activity: current evidence and future directions. *Ann Behav Med.* 1994;16:12-23.
4. Light KC, Dolan CP, Daris MR, Sherwood A. Cardiovascular responses to an active coping challenge as predictors of blood pressure patterns 10 to 15 years later. *Psychosom Med.* 1992;54:217-230.
5. Shapiro AP. An experimental study of comparative responses of blood pressure to different noxious stimuli. *J Chronic Dis.* 1961;13:293-311.
6. Shapiro AP. Pressor responses to noxious stimuli in hypertensive patients: effect of reserpine and chlorothiazide. *Circ.* 1962;26:242-250.
7. Shapiro AP, Krifcher E. Pressor responses to noxious stimuli in hypertensive patients: effects of guanethidine sulfate and alpha methyldopa. *Circ.* 1964;30:671-678.
8. Shapiro AP, Moutsos SE, Krifcher E. Patterns of pressor responses to noxious stimuli in normal, hypertensive and diabetic subjects. *J Clin Invest.* 1963;42:1890-1898.
9. Nicotero JA, Beamer VL, Moutsos SE, Shapiro AP. Effects of propranolol on the pressor response to noxious stimuli in hypertensive patients. *Am J Card.* 22:657-666, 1968.
10. Traub YM, Shaver JA, McDonald RH Jr, Shapiro AP. Effects of practolol on pressor responses to noxious stimuli in hypertensive patients. *Clin Pharm Ther.* 1973;14:165-174.
11. Sapira JD, Shapiro AP. Studies in man on the relationship of adrenergic correlates to pressor responsivity. *Circ.* 1966;34:226-241.
12. Shapiro AP, Nicotero J, Sapira J, Scheib ET. Analysis of the variability of blood pressure, pulse rate and catecholamine responsivity in identical and fraternal twins. *Psychosom Med.* 1968; 30:506-520.
13. Julius S. The blood pressure seeking properties of the central nervous system. *J Hypertension.* 1988;6:177-185.
14. Page IH. *Hypertension Mechanisms.* Orlando, Fla: Grune & Stratton, Inc; 1987:668.
15. Wood DL, Sheps SG, Elveback LR, Schirger A. Cold pressor test as a predictor of hypertension. *Hypertension.* 1984;6:301-306.
16. Menkes MS, Matthews KA, Krantz DS, Lundberg V, Mead LA, Qaqish B, Liang K-Y, Thomas, CB, Pearson TA. Cardiovascular reactivity to the cold pressor test as a predictor of hypertension. *Hypertension.* 1989;14:524-530.
17. Wolf S, Pfeiffer JB, Ripley HS, Winter OS, Wolff HG. Hypertension as a reaction pattern to stress; summary of experimental data on variations in blood pressure and renal blood flow. *Ann Intern Med.* 1948;29:1056-1076.
18. Binger CA, Ackerman AE, Cohen AE, Schroeder HA, Steele JM. *Personality in Arterial Hypertension.* New York: R. Brunner; 1945.
19. Reiser MF, Rosenbaum M, Ferris EB. Psychologic mechanisms in malignant hypertension. *Psychosom Med.* 1951;13:147-159.
20. Reiser MF, Brust AA, Ferris EB, Shapiro AP, Baker HM, Ransohoff WR. Life situations, emotions and the course of patients with arterial hypertension. *Psychosom Med.* 1951;13:133-139.
21. Weiss E, English OS, Fischer HK, Kleinbart M, Zatuchni J. The emotional problems of high blood pressure. *Ann Intern Med.* 1952;37:677-688.
22. Fischer HK. Hypertension and the psyche. In: Brest AM, Moyer JN, eds. *Hahneman Symposium on Hypertension.* Philadelphia: Lea & Febiger; 1961:110.
23. Hambling J. Psychodynamics of sustained high blood pressure. In: *Recent Res Psychosom., Proceedings of 8th Eur. Conf. Psychosom. Res. Psychother. Psychosom.* 1970;18:349-354.
24. Van der Valk JM. Blood pressure change under emotional influences in patients with essential hypertension and control subjects. *J Psychosom Res.* 1957;2:134.

25. Weiner H. Psychosomatic research in essential hypertension: retrospect and prospect. In: Koster M, Musaph H, Visser P, eds. *Psychosomatics in Essential Hypertension.* Basel: S. Karger; 1970:58-116.
26. Holmes TH, Rahe RH. The social readjustment rating scale. *J Psychosom Res.* 1967;11:213.
27. Timio M, Verdecchia P, Vananzi S, Gentili S, Ronconi M, Francocci B, Montanari M, Bichiszo E. Age and blood pressure changes: a 20 year followup study in nuns in a secluded order. *Hypertension.* 1988;12:457-461.
28. Page LB, Danion A, Moellering RC. Antecedents of cardiovascular disease in six Solomon Island societies. *Circ.* 1974;49:1132.
29. Page LB, Friedlander J. Blood pressure, age, and cultural change: A longitudinal study of Solomon Island populations. In: *Blood Pressure Regulation and Aging.* Horan MJ, Srainberg GM, Dunbam JB, Hadley EC, eds. New York: Biochemical Information Corp;1986:11-25.
30. Cassel J. Hypertension and cardiovascular disease in migrants: a potential source of clues? *Int J Epidem.* 1974;224:489-492.
31. Bruhn JG, Wolf S. *The Rosetto story: An Anatomy of Health.* Norman, Okla: University of Oklahoma Press; 1978.
32. Wolf S, Bruhn JG. *The Power of the Clan.* Transactions Publishers: New Brunswick, NJ: 1993.
33. Ruskin A, Beard OW, Schaffer RL. Blast hypertension: Elevated arterial pressure in victims of the Texas City disaster. *Am J Med.* 1948;4:228-236.
34. Graham JDP. High blood pressure after battle. *Lancet.* 1945;1:239-240.
35. Miasnikov AL. The significance of higher nervous activity in the pathogenesis of hypertensive disease. In: Cort JH, Fencl V, He , Jirka J, eds. *The Pathogenesis of Essential Hypertension.* Prague: State Medical Publishing House; 1961:152-162.
36. Henry JP, Stephens PM. *Stress, health and the social environments.* New York: Springer-Verlag; 1977.
37. Gutman, MD and Benson, H Interaction of environmental factors and systemic arterial blood pressure. *Medicine.* 1971;50:543-553.
38. Winkelstein W, Kantor S, Ibrahim M, Sackett D. Familial aggregation of blood pressure. *JAMA.* 1966;195:160.
39. Weiner H. *Psychobiology and human disease.* New York: Elsevier Press; 1977:103-218.
40. Harburg E, Erfyrt JC, Hauenstein LS, Chape C, Shull NJ, Schork MA. Socio-ecological stress, suppressed hostility, skin color and black–white male blood pressure in Detroit. *Psychosom Med.* 1973;35:276-286.
41. Langford HG, Watson RL, Doublas BH. Factors affecting blood pressure in population groups. *Trans Assoc Am Physicians.* 1968;81:135.
42. Farris EJ, Yaekel EH, Medoff HS. Development of hypertension in rats after blasting. *Am J Physiol.* 1945;144:331.
43. Shapiro AP, Melhado J. Observations of blood pressure and other physiological and biochemical mechanisms in rats with behavioral disturbances. *Psychosom Med.* 1958;20:303-313.
44. Belkin GA, Shapiro AP. Behavioral disturbances in animals: II. effects on blood pressure, pepsinogen and adrenal weight in rats. *Tex Rep Biol Med.* 1956;14:415-423.
45. Leenen FH, Shapiro AP. Effect of intermittent electric shock on plasma renin activity in rats. *Proc Soc Exp Biol Med.* 1974;146:534-535.
46. Sapira JD, Lipman RL, Shapiro AP. Hyperresponsivity to angiotensin induced in rats by behavioral stimulation. *Proc Soc Exp Biol Med.* 1966;123:52-55.
47. Shapiro AP, Melhado J. Factors affecting the development of hypertensive vascular disease in rats after renal injury. *Proc Soc Exp Biol Med.* 1957;96:619-623.
48. Lipman RL, Shapiro AP. Effects of behavioral stimulus on blood pressure of rats with experimental pyleonephritis. *Psychosom Med.* 1967;29:612-620.
49. Dahl L, Knudsen KD, Heine M., Leitl G. Hypertension and stress. *Nature (Lond.).* 1968;219:735.
50. Friedman R, Dahl LK. The effect of chronic conflict on the blood pressure of rats with a genetic susceptibility to experimental hypertension. *Psychosom Med.* 1975;37:402-416.

51. Friedman R, Iwai J. Dietary sodium, psychic stress, and genetic predisposition to genetic hypertension. *Proc Soc Exp Biol Med.* 1977; 155:449-452.
52. Folkow B, Hallback M, Lundgren Y, Sivertsson R, Weiss L. Importance of adaptive changes in vascular design for establishment of primary hypertension, studied in man and in spontaneously hypertensive rats. *Circ Res.* 1973;32(suppl to No. 1):I2-I5.
53. Benson H, Herd JA, Morse WH, Kelleher RT. Behavioral induction of arterial hypertension and its reversal. *Am J Physiol.* 1969;217:30.
54. Forsythe R. Blood pressure responses to long-term avoidance schedules in the restrained rhesus monkey. *Psychosom Med.* 1969;31:300-309.
55. Henry JP, Meehan JP, Stephens PM. The use of psychosocial stimuli to induce prolonged systolic hypertension in mice. *Psychosom Med.* 1967;29:408-432.
56. Henry JP, Stephens PM, Santisteban GA. A model of psychosocial hypertension showing reversibility and progression of cardiovascular complications. *Circ Res.* 1975;36:156-164.
57. Henry JP, Liu YY, Nadra WE, Qian CG, Mormede P, LeMaire V, Ely D, Hendley ED. Psychosocial stress can induce chronic hypertension in normotensive strains of rats. *Hypertension.* 1993;21:714-723.
58. Shapiro AP, Horn P. Blood pressure, pepsinogen and behavior in cats subject to experimental production of anxiety. *J Nerv Ment Dis.* 1955;122:222-231.
59. Anderson DE, Kearns WD, Better WE. Progressive hypertension in dogs by avoidance conditioning and saline infusion. *Hypertension.* 1983;5:286-291.
60. Anderson DE, Dietz JR, Murphy P. Behavioural hypertension in sodium loaded dogs is accompanied by sustained sodium retention. *J Hypertension.* 1987;5:99-105.
61. Haythornthwaite JA, Pradley RE, Anderson DE. Behavioral stress potentiates the blood pressure effects of a high sodium intake. *Psychosom Med.* 54:231-239.
62. Gaskell JR, Jones RK, Shapiro AP. Hyperresponsiveness of renal hypertensive rats to intravenous angiotensin II. *Proc Soc Exp Bio Med.* 1964;115:179-182.
63. Sanders BJ, Lawler JE. The borderline hypertensive rat (BHR) as a model for environmentally-induced hypertension: A review and update. *Neurosci & Biobehav Rev.* 1992;16:207-217.
64. Lawler JE, Naylor SK, Abel MM, Baldwin DR. A chronic high-salt diet fails to enhance blood pressure reactivity to a tone associated with footshock in SHR, BHR, and WKY rats. *Physiol and Behav.* 1993;54:941-946.
65. Gelsema AJM, Schoemaker RG, Ruzicka M, Copeland NE. Cardiovascular effects of social stress in borderline hypertensive rats. *J Hypertension.* 1994;12:1019-1028.
66. Reis DJ, Doba N. The central nervous system and neurogenic hypertension. *Prog Cv Dis.* 1974,27.31.
67. Reis DJ, Talman WT. Brain lesions and hypertension. In: de Jong, W, ed. *Experimental and Genetic Models of Hypertension. Handbook of Hypertension.* de Jong, W. (Ed.), Amsterdam: Elsevier; 1984:451-473.
68. Nathan MA, Tucker LW, Severini WH, Reis DJ. Enhancement of conditioned arterial pressure responses in cats after brainstem lesions. *Science.* 1978;201:71.
69. Conway J, Boon N, Vann Jones J, Sleight P. Involvement of the baroreceptor reflexes in the changes in blood pressure with sleep and mental arousal. *Hypertension.* 1983;5:746-748.
70. Chalmers JP, Pilowsky PM. Brainstem and bulbospinal neurotransmitters systems in the control of blood pressure. *J Hypertension.* 1991;9:675-694.
71. Doba N, Reis DJ. Acute fulminating neurogenic hypertension produced by brainstem lesions in the rat. *Circ Res.* 1973;32:584-593.
72. Miller NE, Dworkin BR. Critical issues in therapeutic applications of biofeedback. In: Schwartz GE, Beatty J, eds. *Biofeedback: Theory and Research.* New York: Academic;1977:129-161.
73. Dworkin BR, Filewich RJ, Miller NE, Craigmyle N, Pickering TG. Baroreceptor activation reduces reactivity to noxious stimulation: implications for hypertension. *Science.* 1979;205:1299-1301.
74. Dworkin BR, Ebert T, Rau H, Birbaumer N, Pauli P, Droste C, Brunia CHM. Central effects of baroreceptor activation in humans: attentuation of skeletal reflexes and pain perception. *Proc Nat Acad Sci. USA.* 1994;91:6329-6333.

75. Ebert T, Dworkin BR, Rau H, Pauli P, Birbaumer N, Droste C, Brunia CHM. Sensory effects of baroreceptor activation and perceived stress together predict long-term blood pressure elevations. *Int J Behav Med.* 1994;1:215-228.
76. Guasti L, Cattaneo R, Rinaldi D, Rossi MG, Bianchi L, Gaudio G, Grardi AM, Gorini G, Venco A. Twenty-four-hour noninvasive blood pressure monitoring and pain perception. *Hypertension.* 1995;25:1301-1305.
77a. de Jong W, Sitsen A, Petty MA, Krieger EM. Hot plate sensitivity after baroreceptor denervaation and in hypertension (abstract). *Proc Symp Neurogenic Hyp.* Pittsburgh, September, 1981.
77b. Zamir N, Simantov R, Segal M. Pain sensitivity and endogenous opiates in hypertension (abstract). *Proc Symp Neurogenic Hyp.* Pittsburgh, September, 1981.
78. Zamir N, Shuber E. Altered pain perception in hypertensive humans. *Brain Research.* 1980;201:471-474.
79. Rubin P, Blaschke TF, Guilleminault C. Effect of naloxone, a specific opioid inhibitor on blood pressure fall during sleep. *Circ.* 1981;63:117-1221.

3

Variability of Blood Pressure

DEFINITIONS AND EXAMPLES

At the risk of providing an oxymoron, it must nevertheless be said that variability of BP, as distinguished from reactivity is a constant. Even consecutive BP determinations are rarely the same. A colleague of mine, Joseph Sapira, described this variability succinctly by referring to the fact that "there is no such entity as *the* BP," thus emphasizing the differences which occur between successive determinations, particularly when performed by the standard indirect techniques.[1] I would emphasize that we are defining *variability* here as one of the two components of *lability*, the other being *reactivity* as discussed in chapter 2. Causes of such variability are many and can be classified as *methodological*, *physiological*, and *environmental*.

Methodological

Direct BP is determined by intraarterial puncture and recording of the pulse wave by means of a calibrated manometer. Such techniques are obviously cumbersome, subject to damping of the impulse by blood clotting, and impractical for routine use. They have been used experimentally for continuous recording—for as long as 24 hours by some investigators—but by and large have served primarily to confirm the validity of indirect methods.

As discussed in the introduction, indirect techniques were first developed by Riva-Rocci in 1896 and are based on constricting the arterial blood flow with a cuff inflated on the extremity and then noting the pressure at which the flow returns as the cuff is deflated. This can be done either by palpation of the pulse distally, by oscillometric readings or by listening with the stethoscope for the so-called Korotkoff sounds; the latter has become the standard clinical fashion for determinations although palpation can still offer advantages in certain situations and oscillometric readings are used in some ambulatory indirect recorders. The Korotkoff sounds were first described by N. S. Korotkoff, a Russian physician, in 1905 and consist of a series of five sounds or phases that ensue as the constricting cuff is deflated, the first (K-I), fourth (K-IV), and fifth (K-V) being those of importance to the actual measurement of the prevailing pressure. No sound is heard distal to the constricting cuff when blood flow is completely occluded, but K-I is heard as a faint sound becoming gradually louder as the blood begins to flow. K-I represents the systolic pressure and is probably slightly ahead of the perceived distal pulse obtained by palpation and slightly behind what can be recorded oscillometrically. Diastolic pressure is recorded when the sounds become sharply muffled (K-IV) or when they disappear entirely (K-V) as the blood flow again becomes continuous. There has been continuous controversy in the literature as to whether K-IV or K-V best represents the diastolic pressure. Whereas comparisons with direct arterial measurements suggest that K-IV may be more accurate, it is generally accepted that recognition by the observer of complete disappearance of sound is easier and more reliable than perception of muffling that is somewhat subjective, and hence in the United States at least the use of K-V for diastolic determinations has become standard. One source of error, however, is the problem one experiences in individuals with hyperactive or bounding pulses in which sounds can continue to be heard for longer than the few mm Hg usually separating K-IV and K-V. In these circumstances, it is recommended that both phases be recorded with the true value probably lying somewhere between them.

One of the major causes of methodological error is the difference between the acoustic abilities of different observers that can arise through problems with acuity, carelessness, or patience. This problem can be controlled by training of observers using various types of tapes, at least in research studies in which uniformity is most desired. The speed of the deflation of the cuff will also influence the determination; too rapid a drop can cause the observer to miss initial readings for systolic and fail to note the muffling-disappearance characteristics of K-IV and K-V. There is also the phenomenon of the "auscultatory gap," which is produced by a fading and even disappearance of the systolic sounds during the K-II period and occurs for reasons that may relate to trapping of blood in the venous compartment of the arm.[2] When present it will lead to an underestimation of the systolic pressure when the cuff is not pumped up sufficiently high. It can be detected when a radial pulse is present in spite of the absence of Korotkoff sounds. A more significant problem, however, which can lead to an over estimation of systolic pressure is that noted in the elderly individual with an atherosclerotic, "stiff," brachial artery; in this situation, additional pressure must be applied to the cuff in order to constrict the thickened artery so that SBP will be measured at a higher level than the pressure required to only occlude blood flow. Detection of this phenomenon is accomplished by what has been called Osler's maneuver, namely that palpation of the radial pulse will yield a lower pressure than auscultation of K-I.[3]

A great deal of attention has been given to the width of the cuff and it is now generally standardized that this width should be 15 cm. for general use in most adults. However, it is also clearly recognized that a standard cuff will give a falsely high estimation in an individual with an obese arm, up to as much as 50 mm Hg, because some of the pressure used to occlude the artery is being "wasted" on compacting the soft tissue between the skin and the artery. By the same token, a standard cuff in a child or in an emaciated adult can give a falsely low determination.

The position of the arm relative to the level of the heart can also play a small role in affecting accuracy of the determination. If the arm is elevated, the pressure will be falsely low; if depressed, it will be slightly high. Accordingly, position should be kept constant when repeated readings are being made.[1,4]

Physiological

Diurnal influences are major causes of variability but are often difficult to separate from the effect of environmental stimuli during the day. Usually, when the individual is relaxed and at rest the pressure will fall but the main influence is sleep when both systolic and diastolic pressures may drop 10% to 15% and then rapidly rise to their usual levels when the person awakes. The sleep decline has been known for many years but continuous monitoring in recent studies with ambulatory indirect recorders has considerably increased our observation and understanding of this phenomenon. It is of interest that disorders that affect sympathetic innervation will decrease and even eliminate this nocturnal decline.[5] Thus, individuals with idiopathic postural hypotension of various types will lose their nocturnal fall even when they are normotensive or hypertensive when recumbent during the day. Diabetic patients, even when other signs of autonomic neuropathy are not obvious, show moderate to marked loss of this nocturnal "dipping" often associated with failure of heart rate to fall as well, this latter suggesting a relationship of the loss of nocturnal decline to a maintained relative rapidity of the HR due to vagal impairment as well as sympathetic neuropathy. A most interesting cause of loss of nocturnal decline has been noted in patients who have had cardiac transplantation. Such patients have an autonomically denervated heart in place, HR declines less when they sleep and BP fails to decline and may actually rise above basal levels during the sleep period.[6] Particularly because a majority of heart transplant patients have mild to moderate hypertension, this failure to dip at night may have adverse consequences and at the least complicates the pharmacological management of their hypertension. Similarly, the lack of nocturnal decline at night complicates the management of the diabetic with hypertension and is suggested as one of the reasons for more detrimental effects of hypertension in the diabetic than in the nondiabetic.[7] Long-term studies of the impact of the presence, absence, and magnitude of this nocturnal effect on the course of hypertensive disease in general are needed and remain to be done.

There is normally a small fall in systolic and a slight rise in diastolic along with an increase in HR when an individual rises from the recumbent to the standing position, but the mean blood pressure stays the same. Vasoconstriction and sympathetic outflow to the heart maintain the pressure as blood tends to pool in the lower part of the body. As indicated earlier, some individuals have impaired autonomic innervation that exaggerates the postural fall. Medications that are used to treat hypertension can similarly cause postural fall, both by affecting the ANS or by depleting circulating volume. Accordingly, BP should always be recorded in both recumbent and standing positions on initial examination of a patient and regularly when they are receiving drug therapy. In the sitting position, which is that in which most pressures are routinely taken clinically by most observers, it should be recognized that the pressure is probably closer to that obtained when standing, rather than when recumbent, which however, may be of lesser importance in epidemiological investigations than in the patient management situation.

There is some old evidence to the effect that BP may rise slightly in the hours after a meal and studies with monitoring devices may elucidate these but they are of relatively minor importance.[8] On the other hand, in elderly individuals, postural fall in BP may be exacerbated after meals.[11] What is quite striking however is the marked rise that can occur in BP due to bladder distension.[9] In our own experience, while monitoring patients over several hours in the laboratory during reactivity studies, we have frequently been able to recognize the need of the patient to urinate by otherwise unexplained elevations of 10 to 20 mm Hg, while others who have studied the phenomenon extensively report rise of over 50 mm Hg particularly in individuals with spinal cord injuries.

Environmental

Under the heading of environmental effects on blood pressure, we will discuss both physical and behavioral stimuli. This is to some extent determined by our conviction that these sources cannot be clearly separated and in any case tend to merge with each other. In addition, stimuli that come from "outside" to affect BP must be processed at least initially through the brain and its neural pathways whether they be physical or behavioral and whether they are ultimately expressed peripherally either by a neurological, hormonal, or peptide mediator. Thus, environmental effects influence lability both through the *variability* and the *reactivity* components defined earlier.

One of the most consistent influences on the level of blood pressure is the setting in which the measurement is made. Thus, pressures taken in a medical setting (e.g., in the physician's office or clinic) are almost invariably higher then those taken at home, in neutral surroundings, or by neutral observers. This phenomenon has long been known and a variety of techniques have been employed to circumvent it so as to obtain more reliable measures for both research and clinical reasons. Sir George Pickering in his classic book on high blood pressure in 1955,[10] reviewed some of the investigations pertinent to this aspect of blood pressure variability and his son, Thomas Pickering has popularized the concept in recent years, giving it its current title of "White Coat Hypertension" and exploring its magnitude and frequency with indirect ambulatory recordings.[12] George Pickering described some of his own experiments with Hamilton, Roberts, and Sowry,[13] in which 50% of a randomly selected group of outpatients showed a lower level of pressure on a revisit to the clinic, a phenomenon well known to most clinicians although often a cause of anxiety to both them and to the patient. G. Pickering reviewed some of the even earlier studies of this effect, including Diehl and Lees in 1929[14] who measured blood pressure in 100 healthy medical students every 5 minutes for an hour. They noted that the pressure fell over the first three readings, varied until the 8th reading, which was the lowest, and then slowly rose by the 12th measurement. This observation provides the background to the use of the average of the first three to five readings as the baseline pressure for many of the laboratory studies of stress done by various investigators. In our studies of this type in Cincinnati and Pittsburgh in the 1950s and 1960s we generally took five pressures at 1-minute intervals and averaged the last three. G. Pickering also recalled the studies of Ayman and Goldshine in 1940 in which these investigators looked at home and clinic pressures in a series of patients and found them all lower at home, with a difference of at least 20 mm Hg in diastolic pressure in 24% of the subjects;[15] this observation has been "rediscovered" many times in the last 50 years.

The use of 24-hour indirect ambulatory BP monitors (ABPM) in clinical situations has allowed for a much greater understanding of these environmental impacts on BP. T. Pickering, among others, has defined the "white coat hypertensive" as the individual who has a casual office or clinic pressure that is at the hypertensive level (e.g., 140/90 mm Hg or above) and is normotensive throughout the day with an average level that is below that defined as hypertensive. By these criteria, T. Pickering has reported the existence of this syndrome in as many as 20% of apparent hypertensives as seen in the clinic; others have similarly noted it in the range of 10% to 25%.[16,17] Our own somewhat anecdotal observations, although based on more than 500 ABPMs done clinically over the last 6 years, reveal at least this many individuals who display the syndrome and among them are some in whom repeated measurements have indicated persistence of the phenomena without clinical progression of hypertensive disease over this period of time. Even when they are established hypertensives, we and others have observed that most show their highest pressure when the apparatus is first applied in the clinic with significantly lower pressures during the rest of the day.[7,18]

A large variety of daily events have been noted to cause intermittent and sometimes prolonged spikes in pressure but these are difficult to collect in any precise fashion because of vagaries and omissions in diary entries and the inability to accurately evaluate the emotional and physical content of the events that the patient reports. Certain activities almost invariably elicit small elevations, such as driving a car and talking on the telephone or interacting directly with a colleague at work or a spouse in the home. We have captured elevations that occur while watching sporting events on television or during startling announcements on the television news. For instance, one patient remained at a persistent elevation of about 10% to 20% for several hours while watching the vivid onset of the Gulf War on the early evening news. An interesting observation in this regard is provided by Bruenn in his aforementioned review of the course of Franklin D. Roosevelt's hypertensive disease and has been further reported by Doris Kerns in her recent book on Franklin and Eleanor.[19] During his Yalta trip in late 1944, an evening was spent watching a new movie about Woodrow Wilson, which included references to Wilson's hypertension, stroke, and disability. The movie so disturbed Churchill, that he left the theater, but FDR stayed on to the end, although visually distraught. Bruenn took his BP when FDR returned to his bedroom and found it to be 230/140 mm Hg, perhaps 30 to 40 mm Hg higher than it had previously been running.[19] It was only a few months later (April 1945) that FDR had the massive cerebral hemorrhage from which he died. Such observations are obviously anecdotal but do confirm the impact of disturbing, exciting, and alerting events on individual disturbances of blood pressure and provide explanations for variability.

T. Pickering and his group at Cornell also studied and described the impact of the workplace on BP.[20] Work stress is about equal to the clinic in producing elevated BPs, particularly when the workplace, for a variety of reasons, is particularly provoking. BPs at home in their studies are lower, once again confirming the aforementioned observations made over the years by many observers. It is of interest that the current recommendations by the American College of Physicians, as derived from the meta-analysis done by Appel and Stasson,[21] are that ABPM instrumentation should not be used routinely even though they agree that there is ample evidence that home pressures are lower than office and clinic pressures and that the latter probably overestimate the prevalence of hypertension. Their argument is primarily based on the cost of the procedure versus frequent careful measurements by well-trained observers and the unreliability of some of the instruments currently in use. However, the latter situation is fast being attended to by improvements in instrumentation and training of those who perform the procedure. In regard to cost, this would perhaps be balanced by the money saved in avoiding inappropriate treatment, frequent changes in treatment, and better monitoring of the amount of treatment necessary if more precise and defined average blood pressures were available to the clinician. We agree with Appel and Stassen, however, that the amount of such savings, from our present knowledge base is somewhat speculative, but it can be determined.

Prediction of the course and eventual target organ injury from hypertension has long been sought but as based on single cuff pressures it is unreliable. Perloff, Sokolow, and their coworkers were perhaps the first to show that predictability of target organ damage (TOD) was better determined by average 24-hour ambulatory pressures[22] and more recently, Parati et al. demonstrated that both average pressure and variability relate to TOD.[23] Parati et al. used direct arterial measurements in his studies, whereas studies by Perloff et al. have been with indirect techniques, as have been most recent series. The variability factor (variance) is perhaps somewhat "variable" itself, at least as measured by standard deviations, showing a lack of reproducibility in some studies.[24] Investigators in this area attribute this failure to the different circumstances under which the BP is measured from day to day as well as the problem of separating out the diurnal, perhaps physiological, changes from those occurring due to the impact of various stimuli during the day, such as position, activity, and so on. Again, this is a result of mixture of variability and reactivity. As more reliable methods of indirect measurement are developed, so that technologically erroneous readings can be eliminated, the application of sophisticated statistical methods may allow a better understanding of the factor of variance in prediction of TOD,[25] as well as the more easily understood average BP, which has been referred to as the "hyperbaric impact or load."

VARIABILITY AND PLACEBO EFFECTS IN THE EVALUATION OF THERAPY IN HYPERTENSION

Variability creates a host of problems in the evaluation of therapy in hypertension, both pharmacological and nonpharmacological. In the long run, outcomes of therapy should be based on TOD, morbidity, and mortality but in the short run, outcomes are measured by the effects on BP measurements and hence the variability of all the types discussed earlier can lead to many misconceptions. The science and techniques of clinical pharmacology have to a large extent been developed during studies of therapy in hypertension and the application of these principles are indispensable to any valid interpretation of consequences of a drug or procedure.

Chief among these problems is that produced by the placebo effect. The placebo effect is a conglomerate of many of the influences on variability that we have already discussed, but most important is the impact of the observer on the patient and his or her expectations, and in turn the expectations of the observer. The effect of the placebo on subjective responses is well-known and was studied extensively by Beecher, LaSagna, and their colleagues more than 40 years ago.[26-28] They in fact reviewed studies by Evans and Hoyle on angina pectoris at least two decades before then.[29] But the "power of the placebo" had been known anecdotally since medicines were first used by physicians and other providers, and indeed it can be said that much of the "success" of the medical profession at a time when there were few drugs that had any specific pharmacologic or biological benefits was probably due to placebo effects as well as the tendency for many diseases and symptoms to subside spontaneously. Beecher performed what would in this era be called a meta-analysis by compiling data from a number of studies from different investigators on the results of placebos in relieving subjective symptoms and arrived at the observation that approximately one third of patients derived benefit from placebo use in a variety of diverse conditions ranging from postoperative pain to anxiety and tension. In fact, his interest in this area was motivated by his observations on the relief of pain by saline injections in combat wounded soldiers during the Korean conflict,[30] an event later popularized by one of the episodes in that long-running TV production, *M*A*S*H*. Nor were the effects of placebo limited to beneficial effects; Wolf and Pinsky demonstrated an incidence of both subjective and objective negative affects[31] (e.g., skin rashes from placebos), while Beecher recorded up to 35 different "toxic" effects in his studies.[28]

These observations have been repeatedly confirmed over the years and it is now well recognized by clinical pharmacologists—although unfortunately not always practiced—that any study that does not employ placebos in its design produces results that cannot be relied upon. There has been some discussion recently concerning the ethics of placebo use and indeed if withholding a known benefit from a patient in a clinical situation for the purpose of gathering data is a consequence of placebo use, it is obviously inappropriate[32] but there are ways to adjust to such circumstances in the experimental design. Claude Bernard has said that

> the scientist is distinguished from the metaphysician and the scholastic by the fact that the scientist is not content with only his subjective idea and his deductive logic, but must proceed to the experimental test to achieve objectivity in his search for scientific truths.

The intuitions that initiate his ideas and the reasoning he employs to formulate hypotheses are products of training, motivations, and hopes. As such they are subjected to distortions by conscious and unconscious forces. But the data he derives from his experiments are intended to correct these distortions and to demonstrate to him and his fellow investigators whether the idea is fact or fancy. And to do the experiment appropriately, he must often employ placebos or their equivalent. Otherwise, to again quote Bernard, "he walks at random and is subject to endless illusions."[33] Such experimentation, particularly in clinical pharmacology, often also requires the use of "blinded" techniques in which the investigator does not know which of several test procedures he or she is observing at the time the tests are manipulated. If there is a human subject who is the object of the study, as is the case in evaluations of drugs, the subject is also kept blinded, the study thus becoming what is now known classically as the "double blind" evaluation.

Placebo effects are not limited to subjective symptoms only, but have been shown to have profound objective effects, particularly on BP which brings us back to the major thesis of this discussion. Both the expectations of the subject under study as well as the expectations of the investigator can influence the degree of BP change that occurs. Since the relationship between the subject and the investigator is perforce a doctor–patient relationship, it is affected by the transaction between the two and the investigator's attitudes will affect the responses of the patient. Such transmissions include the enthusiasm—or lack thereof—of the investigator, the interest or anxiety of the patient being exposed to a new drug, and the demands of the investigator on the patient to follow a strict regimen during the study. Reassurance, hospitalization, gender of the patient, and the investigator, are additional factors which influence this transaction. The phenomenon of the "friendly nurse" recording lower pressures than the more "demanding doctor" is well known as an example of the factors affecting the placebo effect. Changes in approach to the patient may be overt but they may also be transmitted through empathetic cues such as the tone of voice and the facial expressions of the investigator.[34]

Reiser et al. reported a study in which experimenters who differed in professional status and concern with the outcome of the study elicited different emotional responses from the patient. Variations in the responses of the BP were noted that were in turn related to the different reactions of the subjects to the different experimenters.[35] We reported an interesting further example of this phenomenon in a 1954 study of a then new veratrum preparation that had been thought from preliminary uncontrolled trials to have a considerable potential as an oral antihypertensive agent. A double-blind, placebo-controlled study was undertaken and the investigator who was involved in the direct care of the patients was initially quite enthused about the study and impressed by the early results. However, because of certain changes in his own life situation, which could be accurately evaluated and dated, he then lost his enthusiasm for the study but continued it to its planned termination. Significant changes in the hypotensive effects of the drug were noted between the period of initial enthusiasm and the later period of nonenthusiasm. These differences in drug effect, related to the two different periods of the study, were at least of equal magnitude to those due to the pharmacologic effect of the drug per se. The placebos were used as well as double blinding techniques; thus we could separate out the three different components of the BP response (i.e., the effect of the drug, the effect of the placebo, and the effect of the attitude of the investigator).[36]

Hospitalization has been shown by us as well as many others to be a most potent "hypotensive agent." In the time before the development of today's potent antihypertensive agents, hospitalization was a major therapeutic tool. Although rest and sleep—the latter a mainstay of Russian investigators—play a role in this effect, the security of the hospital and the solicitousness of the providers were major components.[37] Unfortunately, in the current hospital climate of brief hospital stays and resistance of payers to hospitalization without defining an emergency and without giving specific therapy, this therapeutic approach can now rarely be undertaken. Hospitalization effects can occasionally be "negative" when increasing anxiety is created in the patient or hostile relationships develop between the patient and the staff.

Placebo reactions can also be "titrated." We demonstrated this in studies in 1965 and 1967 in which a dose run-up with placebo alone was performed during initial studies with alpha methyl dopa, then a recently developed antihypertensive agent. Increments in BP decline were noted in some patients related to the number of pills given to the patient, which were assumed by both the patients and nurses to be the active drug.[38,39] Thus, placebo effects are real, potent, both positive and negative, and can be manipulated. Of further interest is the fact that contrary to what may have been anticipated in the early days of placebo use, informing the patient that he or she will be getting a placebo at some phase of the study does not inhibit the effect.

Placebo use is essential to accurately determine the efficacy, and indeed the safety, of new antihypertensive agents. When placebos are not used, extravagant claims as to the value of the new agent appear in the literature and/or in drug company brochures. Ethicists who argue against use of placebos because they may prevent a patient from deriving benefits should be aware of the fact that the placebo treatment may prevent the patient from being harmed by a new drug. Recent criticisms of delay in release of new drugs without adequate clinical trials may be appropriate in devastating diseases without known therapy (e.g., AIDS) but are inappropriate in our opinion when evaluating new drugs to treat BP when so many are currently available. Nor does the placebo-receiving patient need to be "deprived" of active treatment; designs are available or can be developed in which older and established agents are used as a background to which the new drug under study is added, particularly in a more severe hypertensive in whom delay of any therapy at all might be harmful.

In summary, variability complicates our management of patients in therapy and our evaluation of new therapies, but techniques are in place for minimizing those complications, and affording clinicians and investigators challenges and solutions to existing and future problems.

REFERENCES

1. Sapira J. *The art and science of bedside diagnosis.* New York: Urban and Schwarzenberg; 1990: 87.
2. Ibid. p. 92.
3. Messerli F. Osler's maneuver, psuedohypertension and true hypertension in the elderly. *Am J Med.* 1968;80:906-910.
4. Reeves RA. Does this patient have hypertension? How to measure blood pressure. *JAMA.* 1985;273:1211-1218.
5. Mann S, Altman DG, Raftery EB, Bannister R. Inverted daily blood pressure pattern in autonomic impairment. In: *Proceedings of the 9th Annual Meeting of the International Society of Hypertension,* Mexico City, 1982; 267.
6. Reeves RA, Shapiro AP, Thompson ME, Johnsen AM. Loss of nocturnal decline in blood pressure after cardiac transplantation. *Circ.* 1986;73:401-408.
7. Shapiro AP, Karschner JK, Glunk DJ, Barnhill BM. Clinical use of ambulatory blood pressure monitoring: A review of value in patient care. Assessment of diurnal changes related to diabetes, age, gender, and level of blood pressure. *Arch Fam Med.* 1995;4:691-696.
8. Pickering GW. *High blood pressure.* New York: Grune & Stratton, 1955:24.
9. Ibid, pp. 27-28.
10. Ibid, pp. 204-220.
11. Jansen RW, Connelly CM, Kelley-Gagnon MM, Parker JA, Lipsitz MA. Post-prandial hypotension in elderly patients with unexplained syncope. *Arch Intern Med.* 1995;155:945-952.
12. Pickering TG. Blood pressure measurement and detection of hypertension. *Lancet.* 1994;344:31-35.
13. Hamilton M, Pickering GW, Roberts JAF, Sowry GSC. The etiology of essential hypertension. 4. The role of inheritance. *Clin Sci.* 1954;13:273.
14. Diehl HS, Lees HD. Variability of blood pressure. II. A study of systolic pressure at five minute intervals. *Arch Intern Med.* 1929;44:229.
15. Ayman D, Goldshine AD. Blood pressure determinations by patients with essential hypertension: Difference between clinic and home readings before treatment. *Am J Med Sci.* 1940;200:465.
16. Pickering TG, James CD, Boddie C, Harshfield GA, Blank S, Laragh JH. How common is white coat hypertension. *JAMA.* 1988;259:225-228.
17. Myers MG, Oh PI, Reeves R, Joyner CD. Prevalence of white coat hypertension in treated hypertensive patients in the community. *Am J Hyp.* 1995;8:591-597.
18. Prasad N, MacFadyen RJ, Ogston SA, MacDonald TM. Elevated blood pressure during the first two hours of ambulatory blood pressure monitoring: A study comparing consecutive twenty-four-hour monitoring periods. *J Hypertension.* 1995;13:291-295.
19. Goodwin DK. *No ordinary time.* New York: Simon & Schuster;

1994:545.

20. Pickering TG. Ambulatory blood pressure monitoring in clinical practice. *Clin Card.* 1991;14:557-562.
21. Appel LJ, Stasson WB. Ambulatory blood pressure monitoring and blood pressure self-measurement in the diagnosis and management of hypertension. *Ann Intern Med.* 1993;11:867-882.
22. Perloff D, Sokolow M, Cowan RM, Juster RP. Prognostic value of ambulatory blood pressure measurements: Further analyses. *J Hypertenson.* 1989;7:S3-S10.
23. Parati G, Pomidossi G, Albini F, Malaspina D, Mancia G. Relationship of 24 hour blood pressure mean and variability to severity of target organ damage in hypertension. *J Hypertension.* 1987;5:94-98.
24. Reeves RA, Myers MG. Reproduceability of ambulatory blood pressure and assessing treatment withdrawal in hypertension trial. *Am J Hyper.* 1993;6:2923.
25. Verdecchia P, Porcellat C, Schillaci G, Borgioni C, Ciucci A, Battistelli M, Guerrieri M, Gatteschi C, Zampi I, Santucci A, Santucci C, Reboldi G. Ambulatory blood pressure: an independent predictor of prognosis in essential hypertension. *Hypertension.* 1994;4:793-801.
26. Beecher HK, Keats AS, Mostellar F, Lasagna L. The effectiveness of oral analgesics and the problem of placebo "reactors" and "non-reactors." *J Pharm & Exp Therap.* 1953;109:393.
27. Beecher, HK. The powerful placebo. *JAMA.* 1955;159:1602.
28. Beecher HK. Placebos and the evaluation of the subjective reponse. In: Waife SO, Shapiro AP, eds. Clinical Evaluation of New Drugs. New York: Paul B. Hoeber, Inc.; 1959:61-75.
29. Evans W, Hoyle C. The comparative value of drugs used in the continuous treatment of angina pectoris. *Quart J Med.* 1933;2:311.
30. Beecher HK, Deffer PA, Fink FF, Sullivan DB. Field use of methadone and levo-iso-methadone in a combat zone (Hamburg-Hungnam, North Korea). *U.S. Armed Forces M J.* 2:1269, 1951.
31. Wolf S, Pinsky RH. Effects of placebo administration and occurrence of toxic reactions. *JAMA.* 1954;155:339.
32. Rothman KJ, Michales KB. Sounding board: The continuing unethical use of placebo controls. *NEJM.* 1995;331:394-398.
33. Bernard, C. *An introduction to the study of experimental medicine.* New York. Henry Schuman, Inc.; 1949.
34. Shapiro, AP. The Investigator Himself. In: Waife, SO, Shapiro AP, eds. Clinical Evaluation of New Drugs. New York: Paul B. Hoeber, Inc.; 1959:110-119.
35. Reiser MF, Reeves RB, Armington J. Effect of variations in laboratory procedure and experimenter upon the Ballistocardiogram, blood pressure, and heart rate in healthy young men. *Psychosom Med.* 1955;17:185-199.
36. Shapiro AP, Myers T, Reiser MF, Ferris EB. Comparison of blood pressure response to veriloid with that to the doctor-patient relationship. *Psychosom Med.* 1954;15:478-488.
37. Shapiro AP. The influence of emotional variables in the evaluation of hypotensive agents. *Psychosom Med.* 1955;17:291-305.
38. Krifcher E, Moutsos S, Shapiro AP. Comparative studies of methyldopa and placebo in hospitalized hypertensive patients. *Am J Card.* 1965;16:552-561.
39. Moutsos SE, Sapira JD, Scheib ET, Shapiro AP. An analysis of the placebo effect in hospitalized hypertensive patients. *Clin Pharmacol Ther.* 1967;8:676-683.

4

The Hypertensive Personality: A Physiologic and Psychologic Reconciliation

Lability of blood pressure, with its two components of *reactivity* and *variability* as have been defined earlier, may provide the mechanisms by which stress induces hypertension. This hypothesis, however, fails to account for the fact that all of us are similarly subjected to these stimulations yet only 15% to 20% of our species develop hypertension. To deal with this problem, two explanations can be offered. One of these is *quantitative*, namely the frequency and the intensity of the stimuli are the determining factors. Accordingly, those individuals who are exposed to prolonged and repeated stress in their emotional life, their occupational endeavors, and their interpersonal relationships are most likely to develop hypertensive disease. The second sequence is *qualitative*, namely the sensitivity/vulnerability of the pressor mechanisms of the particular individual determines the outcome. Thus, those persons with the more pronounced reactions because of genetic configuration, acquired cardiovascular and renal risk factors, gender, race, and diet, are most prone to consequent hypertension. Much of the research and theorizing about stress and hypertension, as was reviewed in previous chapters and is discussed later, comprise efforts to elucidate this enigma.

PSYCHOANALYTIC CONCEPT

However, there is a third aspect to the psychological considerations in hypertension, one that historically has been prevalent for many years although largely neglected and ignored by present day behaviorists. This is the concept of the particular personality of the potential or actual hypertensive individual, a behavior that derives from the traumas, rewards, and punishments of one's own psychodynamic development. Basically a psychoanalytic concept, this psychodynamic construct produces a pattern of behavior typified by an inability to express hostility and anger in the face of confrontation. The theory then goes on to propose that such energies are channeled through the ANS to exert repetitive stimulation of the pressor mechanisms leading eventually to the development of hypertensive disease. This concept of the hypertensive personality, originally developed by the work of psychoanalysts such as Alexander, Dunbar, and Binger, has heretofore not fit neatly into present day constructs based on reactivity and variability.

The basic premise of the studies by these clinicians was that hypertensives were individuals who were inhibited in their expression of anger and had a need to please others in their interpersonal relationships. Dunbar put it succinctly in 1943[1]

> These patients have had a life-long conflict in the sphere of authority....They have a tendency to feel that the criticisms of the superior are completely unjust although they dare not express their resentment. Their behavior is characterized outwardly as a desire to please combined with chronic rebellion. The typical formula often expressed in just these terms is: "I always have to give in but afterwards I am furious." (p. 264)

Alexander, in particular and Binger proposed that this inhibited anger was then "inwardly directed" and expressed through the autonomic nervous system to produce chronic cardiovascular stimulation, pressor responses, and eventual hypertension.[2,3] In more recent writings, hypertensives have been described as submissive, retreating from confrontation, and displaying problems in tasks requiring active coping.[4,5] Some evidence has been developed that hypertensive patients with more hostility may have more reactivity, and that tasks requiring active engagement evoke greater response than passive conditions.[6] Pertinent to the question of reactivity is the work of Safar et al. in which a change in personality seemed to correlate with a change in hemodynamics as hypertension appeared and progressed.[7] In any case, although investigators have consistently found this pattern of behavior evident in hypertensive subjects, that it initiates a causal nexus, particularly in the sense that Alexander had proposed, has not been established. Nor is it easy to conceive of a prospective experiment that would be feasible and would offer convincing proof of this connection.

An alternative explanation for the particular personality of the hypertensive subject is that at least some behaviors represent *consequences* rather than *causes* of the hypertension. Thus, such behaviors might present as withdrawal from confrontation or suppression of anger, because to react may evoke pressor responses. Second, they might derive from performance deficits secondary to the hypertension per se, which make it difficult to contend with a demanding environmental or interpersonal situation. Data concerning both these sequences are available and I will attempt to demonstrate how the two might be tied together to explain the manifest hypertensive personality, and how in turn the behavior/personality and the pressor reactivity can be reconciled into a unified construct.

Harris et al. and Kalis et al. in the 1950s utilized techniques of psychodrama to demonstrate retreat from confrontation by hypertensive subjects, proposing that this was related to their need to avoid pressor responses.[8,9] Weiner, Singer, and Reiser carried these observations further and observed that when hypertensives were asked to react to the Thematic Apperception Test (TAT), they told relatively uninvolved stories and showed minimal BP responses. When the investigators interviewed the patients and forced increased involvement in the material, pressor responses often occurred. On the basis of these findings, they suggested that hypertensive patients, somehow aware of their tendency to hyperreact, managed to insulate themselves from conflict whenever it was possible.[10]

With Sapira, Scheib, and Moriarty, we investigated this hypothesis further[11] using a pair of movies in which contrasting doctor–patient attitudes were displayed. The movie simulated an office visit of a hypertensive patient to a doctor. In one of the movies the doctor played the part of a gruff and unsympathetic individual, whereas in the contrasting movie he was a gentle and obviously a concerned and considerate person. When these movies were shown to hypertensive patients minimal pressor response was noted, no greater than that seen in a comparable group of normotensive subjects. However, when the patients were interviewed it was discovered that the hypertensive patients denied the very obvious contrasts between the physician demeanors demonstrated in the two movies, whereas the normotensive persons easily recognized the differences. In the course of the interviews, modest pressor responses occurred in the hypertensive subjects that were now significantly greater than those in the normotensive subjects.

These data lend confirmation to the hypothesis that hypertensive persons insulate themselves from situations of conflict. The "insulation" may represent a "behavioral awareness" of innate reactivity (i.e., by failing to perceive a conflict the subject will not react to it and therefore will not suffer the physiological consequences). Such an individual would present manifest behavior in which he or she seems somewhat withdrawn from conflict and unable to express anger and hostile expression in situations obviously calling for it. Thus, this sequence takes into account the observations about the hypertensive personality described previously but turns the relationship around so that the behavior stems from the reactivity rather than the reactivity arising from the behavior.

BEHAVIORAL CONSEQUENCES OF HYPERTENSION

These findings could also be explained if the hypertensive patient had some deficit in perception or processing of stimuli to which he or she was exposed, which raises the question of whether behavioral changes can develop as consequences of hypertension. Over the years, a smattering of reports[12–16] had suggested that this may be the case.

Accordingly, we undertook several years ago to assess a broad battery of psychological functions in a reasonably large sample of newly detected, untreated, young hypertensives and carefully matched normotensive controls. Most information on CNS impairment in hypertension is concerned with major vascular catastrophes (e.g., lacunar infarcts and thrombotic and hemorrhagic strokes). This is equivalent to looking only at irreversible azotemia or hypertensive heart failure as renal and cardiac outcomes of hypertension. Clinicians and investigators, however, are aware of an early fall in filtration fraction (renal blood flow/glomerular filtration rate) and ECG and echocardiographic changes, which are reversible with reduction of BP. Similarly, in our study, when recently diagnosed, untreated and mild hypertensive persons were studied with a battery of tests that measured sensory-perceptual (or "signal input") activities, cognitive (or "central processing") behaviors and psychomotor (or "output") responses, mild but significant impairment of selected functions was noted in all three spheres[17] that were later shown to be at least partially reversible with reduction of blood pressure.[18]

Those behaviors most directly linked to environmental stimuli, such as reaction-time responses, seemed to be relatively less affected than those that were self-initiated or self-cued by the subject. Performance on tasks that placed a demand on both speed and coordination for their successful execution were also reduced below the levels achieved by matched normotensive controls. It is important to note that none of these patients was distinguished by any marked or obvious defect in everyday contacts and it would not appear likely that the deficits that were noted would be intrusive or limiting on ordinary work, family, or avocational activities. These special functional tests impose a load on the subject's ability to respond that, in their way, might be analogous to the use of treadmill pacing for probing more closely into the details of cardiac functioning under stress.

Our observations raised a number of puzzling questions. First, do the deficits reflect a situation that existed prior to the BP elevation; are they the result of something innate to those individuals who later become hypertensive or do they correlate with the presence of increased BP? We have provided some data to suggest that parental hypertension does not contribute to deficits in young normotensive subjects[19] unless perhaps if the genetic trait is marked when both parents are hypertensive.[20]

A second question is whether these behavioral deficits are progressive, becoming more evident with increased duration and severity of the high BP. A third question is whether the deficits diminish when the patients are actively treated for their hypertension. Improvement in function may occur in certain of the behaviors affected as BP is reduced, but it is also possible that specific antihypertensive drugs—particularly those that act through the CNS—may have the effect of aggravating certain deficits while improving others.

As noted above we pursued these questions first in a study in which we investigated the effect of BP lowering in these mild previously untreated hypertensives. Earlier, Goldman et al. reported improvement in one aspect of cognitive functioning in a small group of hypertensives in whom the BP had been lowered slightly by biofeedback therapy.[21] In our work, we were able to retest the majority of our original series of hypertensives and normotensives after 15 months, during which time about half of the hypertensives had their BP significantly lowered by pharmacological therapy, primarily with thiazides. As contrasted with the untreated hypertensives, in whom BP was not significantly reduced, the improvement in the treated patients was greater on 12 of the 15 tests in our battery. In the untreated patients, performance was further impaired in 7 of the 15 tests. Although normal controls showed some improvement, perhaps related to practice and repetition, the rate of improvement in the treated patients was greater in 10 of the 15 tests. When the data were subjected to a *z* score analysis, a highly significant beneficial result was noted in the overall battery of tests in the treated subjects.[18]

Treatment in the group of mildly hypertensive patients described previously was usually with diuretics, which primarily act through peripheral, rather than central mechanisms. Whether drugs that lower BP by other mechanisms cause increments or decrements in performance remains to be studied. The side effects of centrally acting antihypertensive drugs in particular are not well understood at this time. Because there has been increasing attention given to "quality of life" considerations in patients receiving antihypertensive agents, such studies are of major importance. The use of the objective testing of behavioral functions, other than only measures of subjective mood and affect would add much to such analyses.

What are required are carefully controlled, rigorous, prospective studies that will specify extent and type of behavioral effects of central and peripherally acting antihypertensive drugs. Such studies may ultimately make it possible to rank order the available antihypertensive agents with regard to their behavioral expectations, and their potential for other physical side effects, as well as their BP effects, in a fashion that may allow the clinician to make more rational treatment decisions. We are currently engaged in a lengthy analysis of this latter set of questions, and will review the data in detail in the next chapter.

A final question is under what circumstances of severity and duration the deficits may no longer be reversible. In addition, we have provided data that the age of the patient interacts with hypertension to produce deficits,[22] as has previously been shown by Wilkie and Eisdorfer.[23]

As noted previously, the extent and nature of the performance deficits we have described are not detectable by the casual observer nor are they such as to intrude on everyday activities. Suboptimal performance on standardized behavioral tests can be found in a variety of other conditions as, for example, sleep deprivation, alcohol intake, and probably other illnesses. Nevertheless, any chronic impairment of intellectual, perceptual, or psychomotor function, particularly over extended periods of time, can be considered undesirable and to the extent that such changes exist in the individual with hypertension, provide another argument for antihypertensive treatment.

SYNTHESIS OF REACTIVITY/VARIABILITY AND PERSONALITY HYPOTHESES

Reconciliation of the observations and controversies concerning the behavioral influences on hypertension is difficult. There is ample evidence that reactivity to stimuli is a component of BP lability and maintenance. It is often difficult to separate this reactivity from variability related to diurnal (circadian) influences, posture, and various bodily functions. It is unclear as to whether this reactivity is greater in hypertensives and prehypertensives—either in all hypertensives, only those who are essential hypertensive, or only selected groups of the latter. It is also uncertain as to how or indeed whether, this reactivity, occurring repetitively, plays a significant role in the precipitation and perpetuation of hypertension. A body of evidence exists that the hypertensive individual has a personality pattern typified by behaviors of anger inhibition, passivity, and avoidance of confrontation. This was originally a psychoanalytic concept and it was argued that it developed from early psychodynamic experiences and resulted in a channeling of these emotions to ANS discharge. Our later concept has turned this sequence around and proposed that the behavior develops as a consequence of the reactivity (i.e., behavioral awareness of pressor reactivity results in a pattern of avoidance of those conflictual stimuli that would invoke reactions).

The observations of the presence of behavioral deficits in a number of spheres of performance offers the support to the latter concept. Thus, a hypertensive individual, unable to perform at his or her best in a demanding situation, might tend to retreat from it and/or not fully engage in expression of such emotions as anger in an interpersonal relationship. A hypertensive individual who is slowed, particularly in self-cued behaviors where he or she does not perceive subtle cues as well as others, and whose cognitive processes are slightly impaired may be perceived by others as somewhat different than normotensive persons, or may cope less well with social situations requiring confrontation or expression of hostility. Thus, the manifestation called the "hypertensive personality" may represent, in fact, a tacit recognition of the difficulties in performance that have been measured in tests of CNS function.

If we define the *hypertensive personality* then as a consequence of the hypertension, the nagging question of whether pressor reactivity and variability are more marked or not in the hypertensive and prehypertensive becomes moot because increased reactivity as a cause of the personality profile is no longer a necessary condition. The question of whether pressor reactivity and variability may eventually lead to hypertension, or will aggravate existing hypertension, according to the sequence suggested by Folkow et al.,[24] remains pertinent but does not require them to be increased as a precondition. Any lability, be it reactivity or variability, can be harmful eventually or destructive to homeostatic processes, although factors of intensity, duration, and type of stimulus and the pattern of the responding mechanisms, remain pertinent. Thus, the outcome of reactivity in regard to its contribution to the development of hypertension, becomes a quantitative consideration (i.e., how often the patient is stimulated) rather than a qualitative one (i.e., the particular sensitivity of the individual). In this context, behavioral stress factors become only sources of noxious stimuli and bear on the personality only in the sense that various interpersonal or environmental relationships unique to that person, are more or less apt to elicit a stress response.

We propose that we are dealing with two reasonably separate components to explain the behavioral/psychological aspects of hypertension. On the one hand, behavioral stimuli are representative of other stimuli that stress the homeostatic adjustments that control BP and other circulatory mechanisms to meet the oxygen demands of the organism. Their impact can play a role in the distortions and/or exhaustion of these adjustments that can lead to precipitation and perpetuation of hypertensive disease. Second, given the existence of hypertension, behavioral deficits in certain performance characteristics may develop—through as yet unknown mechanisms that may arise from changes in various aspects of CNS neurotransmission, humoral release, and cellular transport—that appear concomitantly with the hypertension and provide for the manifestation of certain personality traits. It is a CNS functional change that presents itself and it may be reversible with BP reduction. Moreover, this concept is analogous to what we readily accept in other target organs. Thus, hypertension causes changes in renal function, manifested in sodium homeostasis and relationships between glomerlar filtration rate (GFR) and renal blood flow (RBF), and in cardiac function, shown by changes in cardiac output and peripheral resistance relationships, which can progress in untreated patients or be reversed with treatment.

To carry this analogy further, the behavioral aspects of hypertension include both contributions to causation of this multifactorial disease, and to functional and organic consequences of the disorder. Likewise, the kidney can cause high BP (e.g., renal arterial stenosis) and suffer from hypertension (e.g., malignant nephrosclerosis); similarly, the heart can cause high BP through increased cardiac output, while hypertension per se leads to cardiac hypertrophy and heart failure. Similar pre- and postdisease implications can be developed concerning others of the proposed mechanisms in the mosaic of factors that influence the causation and outcome of hypertension. This overall concept perhaps is clarifying and in any case suggests new areas for research, rather than the repetitive studies of acquired and innate factors affecting reactivity that have accumulated in the literature to date.

REFERENCES

1. Dunbar F. Psychosomatic Diagnosis. New York: Hoeber;1943:248.
2. Alexander F. Psychosomatic Medicine: its principles and applications. New York: Norton; 1950.
3. Binger CA, Ackerman AE, Cohen AE, Schroeder HA, Steele JM. Personality in Arterial Hypertension. *Psychosom Monographs.* New York: New York;1945.
4. Weiner H. Essential hypertension. In: Weiner H, ed. Psychobiology and Human Disease. Amsterdam: Elsevier-North Holland; 1977:103-217.
5. Esler M, Julius S, Zweifler A, Randall O, Harburg E, Gardiner, H, DeQuattro V. Mild high-renin essential hypertension: a neurogenic human hypertension? *NEJM.* 1977;296:405-410.
6. Steptoe A, Melville D, Ross A. Behavioral response demands, cardiovascular reactivity, and essential hypertension. *Psychosom Med.* 1984;46:33-48.
7. Safar ME, Kamienecka HA, Dimitru VM, Levenson JA, Pauleau NF. Hemodynamic factors and Rorschach testing in borderline and sustained hypertension. *Psychosom Med.* 1978;40:620-630.
8. Kalis BL, Harris RE, Sokolow M, Carpenter LG. Response to psychological stress in patients with essential hypertension. *Am Heart J.* 1957;53:572-580.
9. Harris RE, Sokolow M, Carpenter LG, Freedman M, Hunt SP. Response to psychologic stress in persons who are potentially hypertensive. *Circ.* 1953;7:874-901.

10. Weiner H, Singer MT, Reiser MF. Cardiovascular responses and their psychophysiologic correlates: a study in healthy young adults and patients with peptic ulcer and hypertension. *Psychosom Med.* 1962;24:477-498.
11. Sapira JD, Scheib ET, Moriarty R, Shapiro AP. Differences in perception between hypertensive and normotensive populations. *Psychosom Med.* 1971;33:239-250.
12. Apter N, Halstead N, Heimburger R. Impaired cerebral functions in essential hypertension. *Am J Psychiatry.* 1951;107:808-813.
13. King H. Comparison of fine psychomotor movement by hypertensive and hypotensive subjects. *Perceptual and Motor Skills.* 1956;6:199-204.
14. Boller F, Vitunski P, Mack J, Kim Y. Neuropsychological correlates of hypertension. *Arch Neurol.* 1977;34:701-705.
15. Goldman H, Kleinman K, Snow M, Bidus D, Korol B. Correlation of diastolic blood pressure and signs of cognitive dysfunction in essential hypertension. *Dis Nerv Syst.* 1974;34:571-572.
16. Franceschi M, Tanereli O, Mercinelli A, Canal N. Cognitive processes in hypertension. *Hypertension.* 1982;4:226-229.
17. Shapiro AP, Miller RE, King HE, Ginchereau EH, Fitzgibbon K. Behavioral consequences of mild hypertension. *Hypertension.* 1982;4:355-360.
18. Miller RE, Shapiro AP, King HE, Ginchereau EH, Hosutt JA. Effect of antihypertensive treatment on the behavioral consequences of elevated blood pressure. *Hypertension.* 1984;6:202-208.
19. McCann BS, Shapiro AP, Whitley B, Manuck SB, Miller RE. Absence of behavioral differences in young normotensive adults as a function of parental history of hypertension. *Am J Hyperten.* 1990;3:225-229.
20. Waldstein SR, Jennings JR, Ryan CM, Muldoon MF, Shapiro AP, Polefrone JM, Fazzari TV, Manuck SB. Hypertension and neuropsychological performance: Interactive effects of age. *Health psychology* (In Press), 1995.
21. Goldman H, Kleinman K, Snow M, Bidus D, Korol B. Relationship between essential hypertension and cognitive functioning: effects of biofeedback. *Psychophysiol.* 1975;12:569-573.
22. Shapiro AP, Nixon P, Miller RE, Manuck SB, Jennings JR, King HE. Behavioral consequences of hypertension: effects of age and type of antihypertensive agent. *J Human Hyperten.* 1989;3:435-442.
23. Wilkie F, Eisdorfer C. Intelligence and blood pressure in the aged. *Science.* 1971;172:959-962.
24. Folkow B, Hallback M, Lundgren Y, Sivertsson R, Weiss L. Importance of adaptive change in vascular design for establishment of primary hypertension, studied in man and spontaneously hypertensive rats. *Circ Res.* 1973;32(suppl 1):I-2.

5

Behavior and Antihypertensive Therapy

As discussed in the previous chapter, hypertension per se produces certain subtle changes in behavior. The changes are in a number of domains including perception, central processing, and psychomotor output. These consequences do not particularly affect ordinary day-to-day activities, at least in an easily recognizable manner, but, as we have proposed, may have a bearing on the development of the so-called hypertensive personality. Moreover, they may be improved or changed when BP is lowered and such changes may vary depending on the drugs which are used in treatment. Muldoon et al.[1,2] have reviewed this area extensively for most classes of antihypertensive agents and have emphasized that although current medications are much more specific in their effects on BP than their predecessors such as hospitalization, placebo effects, and sedation, they have many other effects that are unwanted. Such effects adversely influence both the personal experience of the individual patients and the compliance rates of hypertensive populations. The magnitude of this problem was illustrated in the Hypertension Detection and Followup study (HDFP) in which as many as 33% of the previously untreated subjects complained of side effects that required either change in medication or dosage although most of the patients continued in the study using different drugs.[3,4] In terms of the probability that the suspected drug was indeed responsible for the side effect, the majority were classified as only "possible," whereas only 9% were rated as "probable or definite," but nevertheless concern about this aspect of drug therapy is a foremost consideration in the development of the new drugs to which we are currently exposing the large hypertensive population.

Many of the symptoms reported by patients receiving antihypertensive medications imply effects within or arising from the CNS including fatigue, drowsiness, depression, nightmares, impaired concentration, sedation, and dizziness. In the HDFP, the most common complaints after minor gastrointestinal symptoms were of lethargy, dizziness, depression, and weakness, but it was of interest that many of these complaints were present even before specific therapy was started. With the broad variety of relatively nonspecific side effects reported, it becomes imperative to develop methods of study to properly define cause and effect nexi.

Three techniques have been used: side effect tabulations, quality of life (QOL) questionnaires, and neuropsychological assessments. The first of these involves information gathered from the description and enumeration of symptoms during clinical trials and is useful in clinical practice because the data serve to identify the spectrum and incidence of both anticipated and unanticipated medication effects. The second method, QOL assessment, goes further by determining information on the impact of therapy on patients' lives by soliciting data on the impact of the treatment on general health and well-being. Areas addressed include physical symptoms but also pursue comments on social participation, sexual functioning, work performance, and life satisfaction, again usually elicited by investigator or self-administered questionnaires. Findings from QOL studies suggest that pharmacologic treatment of hypertension does, in fact, alter some behaviors, but the literature is inconsistent with respect to the direction of this effect and only recently has exploration of specific effects of the various types of medications been undertaken.

Although useful in identifying important effects of antihypertensive treatment, the data gathered by side effect tabulation and QOL indices have several limitations. Neither method directly evaluates alterations in functioning nor provides precise information regarding the mechanisms by which antihypertensive medications may affect CNS functioning. Additionally, the validity of QOL assessments generally has been defended on the basis of agreement with other subjective measures rather than on correlated objective observations. A comprehensive prospective QOL investigation of antihypertensive treatment by Croog et al.[5] also administered more objective measures of cognitive functioning in addition to questionnaires; after 24 weeks of active treatment, it was noted that captopril, an angiotensin-converting enzyme (ACE) inhibitor, caused more favorable changes on the general well-being index and associated subscales than did alpha methyldopa, a CNS agonist, and propranolol, a beta blocker. However, parallel results were not found with the objective measures. Memory was not affected by any of the drugs and performance on a cognitive task improved with all three drugs. Finally, QOL assessment techniques perforce rely on perceived symptoms and subjective judgments. One is reminded of the study by Jachuck et al. who queried hypertensive patients, their doctors, and close relatives regarding the overall well-being of the patients since beginning medical treatment.[6] The physicians registered 100% improvement in well-being of their patients, half of the patients felt they were improved, whereas the other half felt they were unchanged or worse, and more than 90% of the relatives rated the overall well-being of the patients to be worse!!

The third research strategy applicable to these issues is assessment of behavioral performance. In contrast to information based on symptom reports and perceptions of life quality, this approach directly evaluates each individual's performance on a variety of task skills, making possible the evaluation of antihypertensive treatment effects on the specific aspects of human performance and information processing. These testing procedures have proven sensitive to behavioral sequelae of other medical conditions such as hypothyroidism, diabetes, bradycardia, and uremia. Moreover, the demonstrations of subtle performance decrements in untreated hypertensive individuals relative to normotensives using behavioral performance testing, which we have described in the previous chapter, certainly encourages the employment of these same techniques in the study of medication effects.

BEHAVIORAL PERFORMANCE MEASURES

The majority of the work involves the measurement of performance with traditional neuropsychological tests, and the remainder assesses performance of more typical daily activities, such as automobile driving or the playing of a musical instrument; the latter measures can be referred to as real-life skills performance. With both approaches, changes in quantified behavioral performance are monitored, and, in the case of neuropsychological assessments, testing procedures are standardized.

Two types of study design predominate that can be referred to as observational and investigator-controlled. Observational studies are conducted by administration of a behavioral test battery to two or more groups of individuals differing in terms of BP, medication usage, or both. No attempt is made by the investigators to manipulate or randomize treatment, or blind the subjects as to the medication. Patient groups are compared with regard to potentially confounding characteristics, and average group performances are then compared. Investigator-controlled studies, in contrast, involve the manipulation of antihypertensive therapy in randomized, controlled trials, with testing typically conducted both before and after active medication or placebo.

To summarize, the results of the observational investigations, as provided by the review of Muldoon et al.,[1,2] are quite mixed and further complicated by a variety of design deficiencies. Given these difficulties, whether an association exists between the pharmacologic treatment of hypertension and neuropsychological performance could only be suspected on the basis of this literature.

In comparison with the observational studies, prospective studies that assess behavioral performance both before and after drug therapy much more directly address issues concerning the sequelae of antihypertensive medications. Again in contrast with the handful of available observational studies, a large number of investigator-controlled studies have been published. Muldoon et al.[1] in their review of original and nonduplicated publications of such investigator-controlled studies, noted that the material comprised contributions from investigators in fields ranging from educational psychology to aviation science. The majority of studies included only one class of antihypertensive medication, which was administered for a short period of time, and used limited neuropsychological test batteries.

Beta-Adrenergic Blocking Drugs (BB)

As stated previously, investigations of the neuropsychological effects of specific classes of antihypertensive medications primarily concerns the BBs. A variety of effects might be expected given the reports generated from clinical experience with BBs (anamnestic literature) as well as from related animal experiments. For example, lethargy and sedation are relatively common side effects, and are supported by EEG evidence of CNS depression, and by several animal models of behavioral depression induced by beta blockade. Accordingly, one may predict that the use of a BB would be associated with lower scores on neuropsychological tests of attention, or perhaps even an overall decline in all performance (due to interference with the ability to concentrate). Similarly, from the clinical reports of fatigue and decreased physical endurance supported by experimental evidence of psychomotor slowing and ataxia, BBs might be expected to retard psychomotor performance. On the other hand, the well-established anxiolytic and tremor-reducing properties of BBs might lead one to anticipate that exactly the opposite would occur, namely, that the administration of a BB would improve attention because of reduced test-related anxiety and distractibility, and that lowered muscle tension would improve simple psychomotor performance.

The reviews by Muldoon et al.[1,2] provide these references, and a summary of the findings of controlled trials of the effects of BBs on neuropsychological performance, according to performance domain, is shown in Fig. 5.1, also from this review. The majority of studies report no BB-induced performance changes, relative to baseline or placebo. Although this suggests that no robust drug effects occur, negative results may also result from use of relatively low drug dosages,

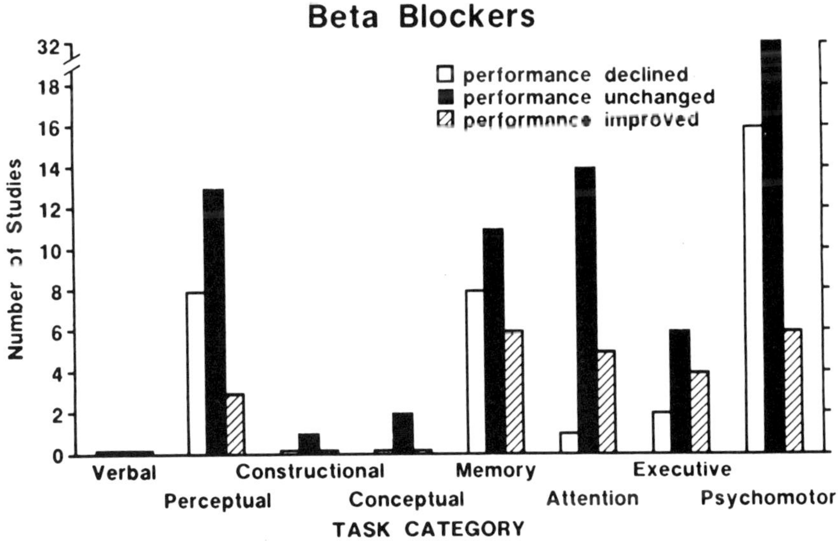

FIG. 5.1. Summary of neuropsychological performance effects of beta blockers in experimental studies surveyed. The data indicate significant differences in performance on medication as compared to control conditions and the marked variability in outcomes in collected studies.

choice of insensitive tests, or low statistical power (many of the studies used sample sizes of 10 or fewer subjects). Within the individual performance domains, no consistent performance decline or improvement was noted. The absence of an observable performance decline on attentional tasks, in reference to the suspected sedative properties of BBs, infers that drowsiness or sedation, if present at all, is either so mild as to not interfere with attention-requiring performance or occurs only in certain individuals. Indeed, the several demonstrations of improved attention with BB usage are in keeping, rather, with an increased resistance to distraction, a byproduct of anxiety reduction. Additionally, the predicted slowing of psychomotor speed with a BB was observed more frequently than increased psychomotor speed.

Several investigations found treatment with a BB to be associated with a decline in perceptual skills, namely an alteration in visual perception, an effect that is not expected from the present understanding of the neuropharmacology of these drugs.

Throughout the literature on the neuropsychological effects of BBs, conflicting findings exist, not only in terms of the presence of a significant effect but even in the direction of effect. This is most clearly illustrated in the domain of memory or learning, in which a roughly equal number of studies report that BBs improve, worsen, and do not alter performance. The inconsistency of findings complicates the interpretation of this literature, although at least a portion of the inconsistent results appears to result from study design differences, including differences in drug dosage, choice of subjects, tests employed, and duration of treatment. No alteration in memory, however, was generally found in studies most closely replicating clinical treatment conditions (i.e., administration of medications to hypertensive subjects for 2 weeks or greater periods of time).

Behavioral performance effects of BBs are generally thought to result from actions of these drugs within the CNS. Given this hypothesized site of action, the degree to which the various members of this drug class penetrate the blood–brain barrier and reach the CNS figures prominently although several authors suggest that psychomotor effects of BBs reflect action on skeletal muscle and that anxiety reduction is the result of peripheral, not CNS, actions.

The major determinant of CNS penetration is lipid solubility, and the BBs have widely varying solubility characteristics. As such, those with greater lipid solubility (e.g., propranolol) appear in higher concentrations within the CNS than those with little lipid solubility (e.g., atenolol). Although questions remain concerning the accuracy of this simple model in chronic drug administration, subjective side effects are often found to be most frequent with high lipid-soluble medications. This, in turn, has led to the suggestion that lipid solubility be used to guide clinical decision making. Whether lipid solubility similarly determines the magnitude of behavioral performance effects of BBs can be addressed by review of those investigations that include two BBs of differing lipid solubility within the same protocol. Such studies suggest that neuropsychological effects are not predominantly a function of relative lipophilicity, because most comparisons found no differences between high and low lipid soluble drugs. However, in those instances in which BBs with differing lipid solubility did produce different effects on neuropsychological performance, it was indeed the lipophilic agent that usually altered performance, whereas the hydrophilic agents tended to leave performance unchanged. Still, the direction of these effects is inconsistent; in comparison with little or no performance effect of poorly lipophilic BBs, ingestion of lipophilic agents occasionally have been associated with improved performance whereas in other studies they are associated with impaired performance.

To summarize, despite the existence of numerous published controlled investigations, the evidence that is available provides little corroboration of hypotheses drawn from related clinical and experimental literatures. Most of the investigations reveal no association of BBs with behavioral performance change. Furthermore, there is no evidence within each of the individual performance domains of robust decline nor improvement with BBs. Relative lipid solubility does not appear to be the major determinant of neuropsychological sequelae, and, finally, exploration of other interactive variables (e.g., drug dose, treatment duration, subject anxiety) has been sparse.

Centrally Acting Sympatholytic Agents

The drug class of centrally acting sympatholytic agents (CASA) includes those medications that lower BP by decreasing efferent sympathetic activity—reserpine, alpha methyldopa, clonidine, and guanabenz. This reduction in sympathetic activity results from either depletion of catecholamine stores (e.g., reserpine) or stimulation of central alpha-2 adrenergic receptors, resulting in negative feedback to catecholamine circuits (e.g., alpha methyldopa, clonidine and guanabenz). Despite reserpine's peripheral site of hypotensive action, it is included with this centrally acting drug class because it also acts within and has side effects referable to the CNS.

In the clinical setting, a clear association is perceived to exist between the use of CASAs and the development of subjective CNS side effects. Uncontrolled investigation and clinical case reports have described disturbances of memory and "mental acuity" in patients receiving CASAs, and prevalence rates of up to 75% have been reported for symptoms such as sedation, tiredness, drowsiness, and daytime somnolence among patients receiving these agents. In the widely cited QOL study by Croog et al.,[5] patients taking alpha methyldopa reported a decline in work performance, whereas those receiving a BB or ACE-inhibitor did not. Experimental studies with animals support these clinical observations with demonstrations, for example, of clonidine-induced suppression of conditioned responding and general locomotor activity. Therefore, one would anticipate that reports of "sedation," "drowsiness," and "fatigue" would be supported by demonstrations of worsened attentional and psychomotor performance in subjects receiving a CASA, and that deficits of higher cognitive skills would be revealed on test performance in the domains of learning and memory or executive functions.

However, the literature on the neuropsychological effects of treatment with CASAs reviewed by Muldoon et al.[1] provides only a few controlled investigations that address this prediction. Although the anticipated association between psychomotor impairment and CASAs was noted in some investigations assessing this type of performance results generally were mixed and consistent evidence for deleterious effects were lacking. In fact, and surprisingly, several investigations reported evidence of performance improvement. Accordingly, with only these few inconsistent investigations on which to judge the actions of CASA, one must conclude that despite frequent clinical reports of CNS-related side effects, little alteration in performance has been demonstrated objectively.

ACE Inhibitors

The ACE inhibitors constitute a comparatively new class of antihypertensive medication; their rapidly increasing popularity is partially due to their reported low incidence of side effects. The mechanism of action of these drugs (inhibition of the formation of the vasoconstricting peptide, angiotensin II) occurs outside of the CNS, and these medications do not appear to cross the blood-brain barrier. Therefore, despite a few intriguing reports of mood elevation, no alteration in neuropsychological performance is expected to result from the treatment with an ACE inhibitor.

Our literature search[1] identified four investigations examining the influence of ACE inhibitors on neuropsychological performance. Drug effects on memory, as well as constructional, executive, and psychomotor skills have been addressed in at least one of these investigations, whereas effects upon other performance domains have received no evaluation. Improved psychomotor performance (finger-tapping speed) with enalapril was revealed in two investigations, one of which also reported a decline in memory. Additionally, executive function was noted to improve in a single report, although no placebo treatment group was included. Hence, with so few published investigations, more definitive conclusions regarding the neuropsychological sequelae of ACE inhibitors requires further research.

Calcium Channel Blockers, Diuretics, and Vasodilators

I conclude this section on the neuropsychological effects of specific antihypertensive medications by mentioning those drug classes whose effects have yet to be carefully studied—the calcium channel blockers, diuretics, and vasodilators (including alpha blockers, ganglionic blockers, and direct vasodilators). Like the ACE inhibitors, the calcium channel blockers and alpha blockers are relatively new antihypertensive drugs that are increasingly being accepted as firstline agents. The diuretics remain extremely popular. Present understanding of the pharmacology of these three drug classes does not suggest they have any action within the CNS. Nonetheless, clinical use of diuretics is associated with an incidence of CNS-related side effects that exceeds that of placebo and their use has been associated with worsened indices of subject-rated work performance and general well-being. In a single controlled investigation of neuropsychological performance including a diuretic, its administration was associated with signs of improvement in constructional and attentional skills, but these findings could well be due to practice effects as there was no placebo treatment group. In a recent, as yet preliminary study, our group has noted some effects on mental flexibility with verapamil, but this observation awaits further analysis,[7] and may apply to other unrelated drugs as well.

EFFECTS ON REAL-LIFE SKILLS PERFORMANCE

In the study of behavioral performance, the measurement of real-life skills performance contrasts in several ways with that of more traditional neuropsychological testing. Real-life skills performance assesses ability in activities more typical of normal daily functioning than neuropsychological testing, and thus any medication-related alterations in performance have more immediate clinical relevance. Again, in being more analogous to daily activities, real-life skills testing may constitute a useful correlate of workplace performance. These theoretical advantages of real-life skills performance over neuropsychological assessment are somewhat offset by their shorter history and therefore less rigorous standardization and validation. Furthermore, most real-life skills require competence simultaneously in several domains of behavioral performance (e.g., musical recital requires memory, psychomotor skill, and auditory perception). Consequently, these measures may imprecisely identify the specific type of cognitive or motor process affected.

In the studies of the effects of antihypertensive medications on real-life skills accumulated for review by Muldoon et al.[1,2] most described effects of a single dose of medication in normotensive subjects. In the remainder, study medications were administered for somewhat longer periods of time, but only two studies enlisted hypertensive subjects. The various real-life skills measured fell into one of five categories: driving or flying, written examinations or proofreading, sports, musicianship, and suturing.

Several interesting observations can be made from this limited sampling. One investigation of the actions of a CASA (reserpine) revealed impairment of driving skills. All other medications under investigation in this literature were BBs; no single instance of real-life skills performance decline was found. Several groups of investigators who have been concerned specifically with the potential for BB-induced impairment of driving or flying skills have failed to demonstrate such deleterious effects.

The pattern of results in two other real-life skill categories suggest that improved functioning may result from the administration of a BB. Several investigations revealed performance on either written examinations or proofreading following ingestion of a BB to be greater than performance following ingestion of a placebo or than predicted by a classroom instructor. Musical performance is another area thta appears to be favorably influenced by use of a BB. First noted in 1977 by James et al.,[8] BB-induced improvement in musical performance (rated by a blinded professional critic) has been demonstrated in most, but not all, subsequent investigations. These findings are often interpreted to reflect the advantageous removal of high sympathetic tone and muscle tension often associated with public performance. From my own clinical and anecdotal information from patients and acquaintances who are performers, I am aware of frequent use of BBs, often without medical supervision, among musicians and public speakers.

MECHANISMS

If little consensus exists regarding the behavioral effects of antihypertensive medications, even less is clear regarding the mechanisms by which these drugs might affect performance. The large number of potential mechanisms reflects the numerous actions of antihypertensive medications. In addition to the variety of peripheral actions on the ANS, kidneys, and vasculature, most classes of antihypertensive medications have other direct or indirect effects on the CNS, all of which can be entertained as potential mediators of behavioral performance changes. Most discussion focuses on the BBs because of the complexity of their pharmacologic actions and the emphasis they have received in this literature.

Via Peripheral Actions

Investigators in this field frequently make a distinction between the peripheral and central actions of antihypertensive medications, and the behavioral effects were first attributed to their peripheral actions. Although these early proposals lacked detailed elaboration on the relationship of the peripheral mechanisms to behavioral changes, an alteration in behavioral performance might result from actions of BBs on neuromuscular function, vascular tone, or striated muscle metabolism. Psychomotor speed and performance, for instance, may be impaired by reductions in either regional muscle blood flow or adrenergically mediated metabolic substrate release. Additionally, motor speed and dexterity may be affected by pharmacologic blockage of beta-adrenoceptors located in the region of the intrafusal fibers of muscle spindles, an activity that may account for effectiveness of BB in treating tremors.

Visceral afferent nerve activity (i.e., autonomic sensory signals of arousal or anxiety) is sometimes considered to be a determinate of performance level. The propensity of antihypertensive agents to alter autonomic activity, therefore, constitutes another mechanism by which these drugs may affect behavioral performance. This model is particularly clear as an extension of the James–Lange theory of emotion, which proposes that emotional stress, rather than being centrally generated and acting downward via the peripheral nervous system, is itself determined by the central perception of incoming autonomic and somatic signals (e.g., pulse rate, sweating, muscle tension, etc.). Therefore, alteration in autonomic activity by antihypertensive drugs may indirectly account for changes in behavioral performance. Eisdorfer, Nowlin, and Wilkie applied this "peripheralist" view in the interpretation of their investigation revealing greater learning task performance and lower free fatty acid levels in elderly subjects receiving propranolol than in those receiving placebo.[9]

Finally, the feature shared in common by all antihypertensive medications is their hypotensive effect, but in our reviews,[1,2] we found few attempts to determine whether the reduction of BP per se is associated with behavioral performance changes. In addressing this possibility, one is confronted with the need to partition the behavioral performance effects of BP reduction and behavioral performance effects of other drug actions (e.g., upon the central and peripheral nervous systems). Nonpharmacologic techniques of reducing BP offer a means to accomplish this separation because there are no additional and potentially confounding drug actions. As mentioned earlier, using biofeedback to reduce the BP of hypertensive subjects, Goldman and Kleinman did demonstrate in an uncontrolled study that BP reduction in hypertensives was associated with improved conceptual abilities.[10,11] In our current work, we have addressed the question of BP reduction and will discuss these findings later in this chapter.

Via CNS Effects

It is the actions of antihypertensive medications on the CNS, particularly those of BBs and CASAs, which receive the most emphasis from investigators concerned with the behavioral sequelae of antihypertensive treatments. The CASAs and BBs bind to a variety of receptors (alpha-adrenergic, beta-adrenergic, as well as serotinergic), which are widely distributed throughout the CNS. Several of the BBs have an additional membrane-stabilizing property. Animal experiments have demonstrated behavioral changes following the administration of BB or CASA to include depression, ataxia, decreased fighting and conditioned responding, as well as physiologic alterations in EEG pattern, sleep cycles, and CNS hormone secretion. A biphasic dose-response function was revealed in the work of Itil and Itil in which 40 mg of propranolol produced an EEG pattern reminiscent of vigilance-enhancing compounds, whereas 80 mg produced an EEG pattern similar to sedative-hypnotic drugs.[12] Our review revealed several attempts to correlate EEG findings during beta-adrenergic blockade with neuropsychological effects in humans, but the results were mixed. Thus, although it is likely that many of the neuronal circuits with which BBs and CASAs interact are involved in processes such as motor coordination, memory recall, or higher cognitive processes, as yet there has been little elucidation of the central mechanisms by which these medications may alter behavioral performance.

The final action of antihypertensive medications that may possibly mediate behavioral performance concerns alterations in cerebral blood flow (CBF). CBF is "protected" from acute alterations in systemic BP through autoregulatory mechanisms involving small vessel cerebrovascular resistance but the stability of CBF during sustained BP changes is less certain. In 1946, Kety and Schmidt[13] described low CBF in a small group of hypertensive individuals, and since that time evidence has accumulated that demonstrates both structural and functional alterations in cerebral circulation, even in untreated and uncomplicated hypertension. Such early vascular changes are manifest in hypertrophy of cerebral blood vessels, decreased common carotid blood flow, impaired endothelium-dependent dilation of cerebral arterioles, and elevation of the lower limit of autoregulation, each of which potentially jeopardize the maintenance of CBF when BP is chronically lowered.

With the institution of drug treatment, changes in CBF may be anticipated because of this vulnerability of cerebral perfusion in the hypertensive individual, and because many antihypertensive medications interact with amines and peptides thought to regulate cerebrovascular resistance. Technical limitations have prevented serial and noninvasive measurement of antihypertensive treatment effects on cerebral blood flow, but the introduction of the Xenon-133 inhalation and pulsed Doppler methods has now allowed their description in a variety of settings. A decline in global CBF may be noted in the acute treatment of hypertension, probably resulting from a reduction in BP below the lower limit of autoregulation. In contrast, cerebral perfusion during chronic pharmacologic treatment of hypertension, appears to be protected since several investigations have revealed that chronic administration of BBs, CASAs, ACE inhibitors, and vasodilators either increases or does not change CBF. Thus, despite lowering BP, many antihypertensive medications do not appear to cause the anticipated decline in CBF. Instead, these results imply that the chronic treatment of hypertension is associated with a concomitant reduction in cerebral vascular resistance. These dynamic changes in cerebral perfusion during chronic hypertension and its treatment need further exploration in relation to behavioral performance alterations. In the near future, the development of PET scanning may offer a more precise method of correlating behavioral performance with CNS change.

SUMMARY AND CONCLUSIONS

In our reviews of the clinical investigations, both observational and investigator-controlled, which examined the behavioral performance effects of antihypertensive medications, we attempted to discern patterns of results that might prove useful in the treatment of hypertension. Despite the sizable number of studies uncovered, only a portion of the neuropsychological performance categories have been addressed and several classes of antihypertensive medications remain virtually untested. A variety of methodologic concerns have also arisen, some of which significantly alter the clinical relevance of this literature.

With regard to the observational studies we reviewed, findings do not consistently show either improvement or decrement in behavioral performance to be associated with the pharmacologic treatment of hypertension. Methodologically, many lack an appropriate comparison group consisting of placebo-treated hypertensives. The numerous investigator-controlled studies have primarily focused on the behavioral performance effects of one class of medication—BBs. Inconsistent and conflicting findings are common and probably result from differences in design of the various studies and interaction with other variables, such as individual differences in anxiety. Although BBs may, in certain circumstances, result in some impaired performance of simple psychomotor skills, little support is found for sedation or decreased attention with these medications. Some preliminary evidence suggests that visual perceptual skills may be impaired. Performance of tasks more similar to real-life activities do not appear to decline with BBs, and musical performance and written examination scores may improve. Finally, none of the behavioral performance effects of BBs appears to be solely influenced by lipid solubility.

The few CASA investigations find, in common with BBs, that there may be some impairment of simple psychomotor skills, but do not reveal further evidence of substantial decremental effects on behavioral performance. Too few investigations have been conducted using the other classes of antihypertensive medications for one to draw meaningful conclusions.

Caution, however, should be used in the clinical interpretation of much of this literature. Throughout our summary of these investigations shortcomings have been apparent that limit the usefulness of much of this work for identifying performance effects of clinical relevance. First, the sample sizes were frequently small, thereby increasing the likelihood of Type II errors. Second, although neuropsychological performance is known to be influenced by a large number of subject variables, few of these factors were regularly addressed when comparing subject characteristics between treatment groups. Third, because most studies were prospective and involved the repeated administration of test batteries, confounding practice effects must be accounted for. This necessitates the incorporation of a parallel placebo-treated group or the use of a random-order crossover design. Numerous studies, however, compared performance in the beginning of the study while off active medications with later performance on active treatment. Fourth, the test batteries chosen were frequently narrow and limited. Finally, very few investigations administered a range of drug doses despite the great importance, from a pharmacologic perspective, of a demonstrable dose-response relationship.

Perhaps more crucial than these methodologic shortcomings, the design of most investigations failed to mimic the use of these medications in the clinical setting. Often normotensive subjects were enrolled to receive single doses of each study medication. It is increasingly recognized that hypertensive individuals, prior to treatment, differ from normotensive individuals in several aspects of neuropsychological performance, and, furthermore, experience different cardiovascular responses to antihypertensive medications. Additionally, little can be extrapolated from the effects of a single dose regarding possible effects of months or years of treatment since tolerance, or its complement, sensitization, may develop over time. However, although a clear majority of the investigations revealed no drug-induced behavioral effects, neither do these data provide credible support for the null hypothesis, due to the methodologic deficiencies and low statistical power of many of the investigations.

Reconciliation of some of the controversies and inconsistencies discussed in this chapter may derive from a study we have recently completed and is currently published in preliminary and abstract form.[7,14] This study was performed in a large group of mild hypertensives (n = 69) who were studied while on three pairs of contrasting drugs: hydrochlorothiazide versus alphamethyl dopa; enalapril versus verapamil; and metoprolol versus atenolol. Blood pressure decline with all six drugs was essentially the same averaging approximately 10/7 mm Hg. A comprehensive battery of neuropsychological tests was performed during each drug period interspersed with placebo periods and a dose run-up was done in those patients who showed lesser responses. The design answered many of the problems we have described earlier in this chapter.

The results of the neuropsychological tests showed a definite impairment in mental flexibility, of only modest degree, and an improvement in functions that measured memory. Because the drugs all varied in their mechanism of BP reduction—hydrochlorothiazide is a diuretic; alphamethyl dopa is a CNS agonist; enalapril is an ACE inhibitor; verapamil is a calcium channel blocker; metoprolol is a lipophilic beta blocker; atenolol is a hydrophilic beta blocker—the drugs would be expected, theoretically and in terms of the data we have discussed earlier in this chapter, to have had differing effects on behavior. The fact that we could not distinguish between them behaviorally but they all reduced BP to the same degree, strongly suggests that the changes in behavior were a function of improvement in hypertension per se. Thus, from this study, in which most of the confounding factors were controlled, our data support the concept that in spite of conflicting clinical observations, both subjective and objective, concerning the behavioral effects of different drugs, the most likely explanation for change is indeed reduction in blood pressure.

Finally, much current controversy, discussed in chapter 6, persists between avid proponents of the "naturalistic" therapies and advocates of rational clinical pharmacological approaches to the management of hypertension. Certainly there is a role for lifestyle change and behavioral considerations in this disease as we have discussed and will further elucidate. But that part of the controversy that is based on the negative behavioral aspects of pharmacological therapy is somewhat overdone. As our forgoing reviews have indicated, the effects of antihypertensive drugs on behavior, although real, are not inhibiting in most instances and broad statements concerning their harmful impact are inappropriate. The problem should not be approached as an "either and or" proposition and behavioral side effects should not be a major argument for the use of nonpharmacological methods of therapy. At the same time, any investigation of a drug, new or old, should include a design that permits gathering of accurate data, both subjective and objective, on the impact of the drug on behavior and real life skills, Thus, the clinician and patient both will know what to anticipate and can make the best decisions concerning when, which, and how to use medications. Such parameters in clinical pharmacological research should be included; much remains to be done.

REFERENCES

1. Muldoon MF, Shapiro AP, Manuck SB, Waldstein SR. Behavioral sequelae of antihypertensive therapy: A review. In: Shapiro AP, Baum A, eds. *Perspectives in Behavioral Medicine. Behavioral Aspects of Cardiovascular Disease.* Hillsdale, NJ: Lawrence Erlbaum Associates; 1991:287-324.
2. Muldoon MF, Manuck SB, Shapiro AP, Waldstein SP. Neurobehavioral effects of antihypertensive medications. *J Hyperten.* 1991;9:549-559.

3. Five year findings of the Hypertension Detection and Followup Program. I. Reduction in mortality of persons with high blood pressure, including mild hypertension. HDFP Cooperative Group, DHEW: (A.P. Shapiro, Chairman, Policy Advisory Board) *JAMA.* 1979;243:2562-2571.
4. Five year findings of the Hypertension Detection and Followup Program. II. Mortality by race, sex and age. HDFP Cooperative Group, DHEW: (A.P. Shapiro, Chairman, Policy Advisory Board) *JAMA.* 1979;243:2572-2577.
5. Croog SH, Levine S, Testa MA, Brown B, Bulpitt CJ, Jenkins CD, Klerman GL, Williams GH. The effects of antihypertensive therapy on the quality of life. *NEJM.* 1986;314:1657-1664.
6. Jachuck SJ, Brierley H, Jachuck S, Willcox PM. The effect of hypotensive drugs on the quality of life. *J Royal Col Gen Pract.* 1982;32:103-105.
7. Shapiro AP, Muldoon MF, Waldstein SR, Jennings JR, Manuck SB. Blood pressure and behavioral effects of antihypertensive medications: A preliminary report. In: Dimsdale JE, Baum A, eds. Quality of Life in Behavioral Research. Hillsdale, NJ: Lawrence Erlbaum Associates; 1995:115-119.
8. James, IM, Pearson RM, Griffith DNW, Newbury P. Effect of oxprenolol on stage-fright in musicians. *Lancet.* 1977;2:952-954.
9. Eisdorfer C, Nowlin J, Wilkie F. Improvement of learning in the aged by modification of autonomic nervous system activity. *Science.* 1970;170:1327-1329.
10. Goldman H, Kleinman KM, Snow MY, Bidus DR, Korol B. Relationship between essential hypertension and cognitive functioning: Effects of biofeedback. *Psychophysiol.* 1975;12:569-573.
11. Kleinman KM, Goldman H, Snow MY, Korol B. Relationship between essential hypertension and cognitive functioning II: Effects of biofeedback training generalize to non-laboratory environment. *Psychophysiol.* 1977;14:192-197.
12. Itil TM, Itil KZ. Central mechanisms of clonidine and propranolol in man. *Chest.* 1983;83(suppl 1):411-416.
13. Kety SS, Schmidt CF. Cerebral blood flow and cerebral oxygen consumption in 5 patients with hypertension. *Am J Med Sci.* 1946;212:124-125.
14. Muldoon MF, Waldstein SR, Jennings JR, Ryan CM, Shapiro AP, Polefrone JM, Manuck SB. Neuropsychological performance effects of antihypertensive medications. *Psychosom Med.* 1996;58:76(Abstract).

6

Nonpharmacological Treatment of Hypertension

The health benefit from lowering BP in hypertensive patients has been a major clinical research accomplishment of the last four decades, one that I have had the privilege of observing and participating in since my early experiences in Cincinnati in the late 1940s and 1950s when our efforts were primarily diagnostic and therapy was limited to reassurance, hope, and prayer. Our pharmacological efforts at that time were concerned with evaluating acute effects of potent drugs such as the ganglionic blocking agents and the veratrum alkaloids and their applications to therapy were limited because of their potent side effects. We were only beginning to emerge from drastic efforts at high BP reduction with such primitive efforts as nitrates, fever therapy, and sympathectomy. We did follow hypertensive patients closely in our clinics and were impressed by the variability of BP and by the value of supportive therapy—mainly reassurance, hospitalization, and lifestyle changes—in reducing BP and even occasionally reversing or delaying consequences of the disease. Reiser et al., in fact, reported a small group of patients in whom malignant hypertension was ameliorated in this fashion, at least for a brief period of time.[1] Nonpharmacological therapy was the order of the day because essentially specific drugs to treat hypertension were not available. Indeed we preferred to speak of the drugs that began to emerge in the 1950s as "hypotensive" agents and not as "antihypertensive" drugs.

Pharmacological therapy of malignant hypertension did make progress in the 1950s with the advent of combinations of long acting ganglionic blocking agents, the vasodilator drug, hydralazine, and the diuretics of the thiazide genre. With these agents, the malignant phase of the disease could be reverted to a more benign course, but their use in the more modest forms of hypertension and in those with mild disease was inhibited by their disturbing side effects that interfered in many ways with patient comfort and lifestyle. Orthostatic symptoms, difficulty in urination, constipation, headaches, impotence—both libidinous and erectile failure—were all very real problems in their use and although these could be tolerated in patients with the malignant and more severe phases of hypertension, it was difficult to justify their administration in the asymptomatic mild hypertensive. There was uncertainty as to whether life expectancy was shortened even in the individual with modest degrees of hypertension (i.e., diastolics of 100 to 115 mm Hg) and it was generally felt that with mild hypertension (i.e., diastolics of 90 to 105 mm Hg, who constituted about two thirds of the hypertensive population, the risk of death and even of significant morbidity was minimal. Accordingly, we felt justified in viewing our approach with reassurance and supportive therapy, often accompanied by admonitions for weight control and a low salt diet, as a method of management. These measures did result in significant lowering of BP as we showed in the aforementioned (chapter 2) studies from our group in Cincinnati in 1951.[2] Beyond the supportive therapy which we offered to our patients, there were reports of significant lowering of BP with more extensive psychotherapy, including psychoanalysis. These now historic events are pointed out to illustrate that the idea of treating hypertension with behavioral techniques is not a new concept, but rather one that was relied on before the advent of current pharmacological treatment.

Over the last thirty years we have come full circle. Pharmacological therapy first showed its value in the nonmalignant hypertensive in the studies of Freis and his coworkers in their classic study in a relatively small group of male patients in the 1960s, performed in a Veterans population, and treated with reserpine, thiazides, and hydralazine. The patients were divided into three groups depending on their BP levels defined as severe, moderate, and mild. A definite diminution in deaths and morbidity primarily from cerebrovascular events was demonstrated in the first two of these groups, namely those with BPs of over 115 mm Hg and those with levels from 105 to 115 mm Hg, but it was still unclear that an appreciable impact was made on the mild group with BPs of 90 to 105 mm Hg.[(3-5)] It remained for the Hypertension Detection and Followup Program (HDFP), a study conducted in 14 centers throughout the United States, which I had the privilege of being involved with as chairman of the Policy Advisory Board, to establish the value of treatment in the mild group. The HDFP enlisted and studied a population of 10,000 patients, recruited directly by house-to-house surveys in selected census tracts who were treated and followed for a minimum of 5 years; it began in the early 1970s and was reported in 1979.[6,7] The design of the study was relatively simple; the patients were randomly divided into two groups, one of which received special care (SC) in clinics especially established for the purpose of goal-oriented, intensive stepped care. Patients were followed closely with medications added as necessary to achieve *diastolic* BPs of 90 mm Hg or at least 10 mm Hg below their baseline. Medications used were reserpine—and later propranolol—thiazides, hydralazine, methyl dopa, and guanethidine sulfate, added stepwise to achieve the aforementioned goal. The other group of patients were assigned to regular care (RC), meaning that they were turned over to their regular source of treatment, usually from their community physicians, but were seen yearly by the investigators for evaluation and followup. The majority of the RC patients also received some therapy from their regular source, but it was not of the intensity or goal orientation of the SC group. Although it was not considered ethical or appropriate to have a placebo group, it was recognized that the RC group would have less intense treatment since, particularly for the mild hypertensives, this was the *Zeitgeist* during this period of time.

The results were impressive. The primary endpoint was overall mortality and there was a greater than 16% decrease in deaths in the SC group and this difference was most marked in the so-called mild hypertensive patients. In fact the differences were less in the moderate and severe patients, a fact that was interpreted as meaning that the physicians caring for the RC patients were more convinced of the need for aggressive therapy in their more severe hypertensives than they were of the need for therapy in the milder forms of the disorder. The major cause of death that was prevented, was again—as in the Freis study—in cerebrovascular events. Evidence for prevention of death from cardiac causes was much less convincing, despite the fact that hypertension is considered a significant risk factor in cardiac, particularly coronary atherosclerotic, disease. The meaning of this failure to demonstrate a decrease in coronary artery disease (CAD) mortality has created a storm of controversy that remains to this day. It has been blamed on poor choice of drugs—although at the time of this study only the ones used were pharmacologically available—electrolyte abnormalities, exaggeration of lipid risk factors, and the additional genetic/environmental/behavioral influences on atherosclerotic CAD, as contrasted to cerebrovascular disease. Personally, we have come to believe that the difference is not due to drug factors but to the fact that the connection between hypertension and CAD is not as direct a one as it is between cerebrovascular disease, particularly cerebral hemorrhage, and hypertension.

These data, along with subsequent clinical trials, have firmly established that treatment of hypertension with present day pharmacological agents has a significant impact on morbidity and mortality of the disease. As pointed out in an earlier chapter, the development, evaluation, and marketing of drugs to treat hypertension has become a major industry whose goal is treatment for most all hypertensive subjects who number some 15% to 20% of the population. At the same time, however, the "pathopharmacology" of these drugs has posed a considerable problem and has led us, as mentioned earlier, full circle to a reconsideration of nonpharmacological means of treatment, particularly in the milder degrees of hypertension. The problem of side effects of drugs is of course not insurmountable; in the aforementioned HDFP study, for example, although about one third of patients reported difficulties with one or another of the drugs they were receiving, only 9% had to be dropped from the program. The rest were successfully transferred to other drugs. Nevertheless, the problem has served as an impetus and a challenge to advocates of behavioral therapies and dietary and lifestyle change as alternative methods of treatment.

Under the heading of dietary changes in management, control of weight and reduction of sodium intake constitute the two major approaches. Calcium or potassium supplementation to the diet have had their advocates. Smoking cessation, alcohol restriction, and physical exercise have been scrutinized as lifestyle changes that can influence BP. Avoidance of daily stress by change in occupation, environment, climatic extremes, spouse and associates, and the like, all have had a long history of being offered as gratuitous advice to patients by friends, family, and indeed by physicians and other health care providers. Control of these factors requires knowledge of the social and cultural forces that influence them as well as the development of techniques to put them into effect, and in this respect behavioral manipulation, defined in a broad way, is essential. But the specific behavioral therapies that have been utilized to lower BP have more direct psychological origins. They include psychotherapy, environmental modification, suggestion, placebo administration, relaxation, and biofeedback. The background, utilization, and outcomes for each of these are discussed. First, however, some discussion of the dietary and life changes is in order.

SODIUM INTAKE

Diet is strongly influenced by social and cultural factors and accordingly is affected by behavior. Most important to the consideration of hypertension is sodium intake and in fact Denton has argued that the salt-seeking behavior of humans has had a major evolutionary impact.[8] Some of the most potent adaptations in humans are directed at sodium control and the phylogenetic development of the renin-angiotensin system (RAS) primarily relates to sodium conservation. Salt is essential to human life, yet its intake can vary from as low as 1 mequiv/day to as high as 400 and perhaps 800 mequiv/day, while the person still maintains normal health and function. Sodium intake has been considered a significant factor in the pathogenesis of hypertension for many years and we do not intend to cover this literature in any detail in the present discussion. However, some of the epidemiological data concerning the effects of sodium are pertinent to the social, cultural, and behavioral influences on hypertension, which are within our agenda. Studies of various cultural groups have indicated that sodium intake in close, primitive societies correlates with differences in levels of BP among such societies. Sodium intake in the most primitive tribes is quite low as is the prevalence of hypertension within them. Cassel[9] and Henry[10] have discussed the process of acculturation in terms of the stress that particular societies experience, but Lot Page[11] has suggested that this process of acculturation is also associated with increased sodium intake which plays an equally important role in their development of hypertension.

The sodium intake of civilized people (150 to 200 mequiv/day) can be considered high and "unnatural" since primitive groups often subsist adequately even in hot climates with intakes of less than 40 mequiv/day. Older studies of the Yanomano Indians of South America have been particularly revealing in this regard; their sodium intake averages 5 mequiv/day and there is literally no hypertension among them and they do not show the BP rise that occurs with aging. It is of interest, in view of what we have said earlier about the evolutionary development of the RAS as a sodium-conserving mechanism that the Yanomanos maintain their low BPs despite peripheral renin activities (PRA) that are two to three times normal values.[12]

In regard to sodium conservation as an evolutionary development, an interesting theory has been put forward by Grim to possibly explain the higher prevalence of hypertension among African Americans in the United States.[13] He argues that Blacks from the interior of equatorial Africa had developed more potent sodium conservation mechanisms than those from coastal areas, and they survived the rigors of the slave trade to a greater extent during the long sea voyages that brought them to this country. Deaths on the slave ships were massive and most were due to sodium-depleting causes (e.g., malnutrition, diarrhea, heat, fever, etc.). Thus, the Blacks in the United States constitute the major descendants of this sodium-conserving group, retaining sodium more avidly, having now a higher predilection to hypertension, and responding more dramatically to sodium restriction and diuretic therapy. Whether such a genetic selection could have taken place in the brief period of the past several hundred years is a matter of speculation but it is an interesting hypothesis that is perhaps amenable to further investigation.

The evidence that a decrease in sodium intake in the diet will lower BP in man derives mainly from the effectiveness of the diuretics and from the results of drastic sodium restriction with such regimens as the Kempner rice diets of years ago, in which sodium intake was decreased to approximately 10 mequiv/day. Direct evidence that lesser degrees of sodium restriction, on the order of 75 to 100 mequiv/day that could be achieved by avoidance of added salt and well-known high sodium foods, can have a measurable effect on BP in humans, is less available. A study by Parijs et al. demonstrated that a reduction from the usual 200 mequiv/day to approximately 100 lowered BP about 10/5 mm Hg and supplemented the effect of diuretics.[14] Similarly, Morgan et al. demonstrated a diastolic decline averaging 7.3 mm Hg in a group of patients with a sodium intake reduction reflected in urinary sodium decrease from approximately 191 mequiv to only an average of 157 mequiv/day. There was a wide variation in the success in reducing sodium intake in Morgan's patients; those with values approaching 100 mequiv/day had the better BP results. These results occurred and persisted over a 2-year period.[15] A recent study of interest, by Singer et al.[16] relates to the additive effect of lowering sodium on the hypotensive effect of an ACE inhibitor. These investigators showed that modest reduction of sodium intake (from 206 mequiv/day to 109 mequiv/day) was equally effective as hydrochlorothiazide in improving BP control.

Luft and his colleagues have derived the reverse data, namely that in healthy people put on progressively high intakes of sodium starting at low levels and rising to as high as 800 mequiv/day, BP will show a proportional rise.[17] This certainly would be expected from animal data like those of Menely and Dahl who showed this phenomenon in numerous experiments over the years.[18,19] Quite striking, however, in terms of Dahl's data on genetic differences in salt sensitive and resistant rats, studies of increased sodium intake reported by Kawasaki et al. noted that mild hypertensive patients divided themselves into groups who were quite sensitive to salt intake and others who were considerably less sensitive.[20]

What does all of this mean as a behavioral or cultural risk factor for hypertension? First of all, we do not really understand our craving for excessive salt intake beyond our physiologic need and our ability to conserve it. It seems at least in part to be a learned habit. There is evidence that infants have little or no taste for salt, a fact that has finally persuaded some baby food manufacturers to remove sodium from baby food products since they primarily were adding it for the "tasting mothers" rather than the "consuming infants." Avoidance of salt can be learned (or perhaps salt taste can be "unlearned") as has been the experience in treating hypertensives; anecdotally, patients who observe this behavior for a significant period of time develop a sensitive sodium taste threshold and can taste salt in situations where others do not.

On the other hand, however, there seems to be some evidence that there is an increased salt avidity in hypertensives. The question "Do you salt your food before you taste it?" is said to be answered in the positive by hypertensive patients although there is no adequately controlled study of this phenomenon that includes normotensives. Interestingly, Langford et al. showed that patients put on diuretics can develop an increased salt intake if they are not closely watched in this regard.[21] This is reminiscent of old observations that demonstrated that sodium depleted rats (e.g., after adrenalectomy) preferentially will consume saline-containing fluid when offered, rather than water alone.

These data suggest that humans have developed a powerful tool to maintain the sodium content and concentration in our bodies at adequate levels for maintenance of life, and this process has played a significant evolutionary role in development from marine to terrestrial animals. This mechanism may have evolved in humans under certain environmental circumstances as per Grim's hypothesis as outlined earlier. Because of cooking and preserving habits and other cultural influences on taste in modern society, we currently consume considerably more sodium than we need for our vital body functions and it is probable that this increase in sodium intake, at least in particularly prone individuals, plays a significant role in *predisposition* and *perpetuation* of hypertension.

Reduction of sodium intake in humans to a more physiologic amount (e.g., 100 mequiv/day or about 4 to 5 grams of salt) would require major social and cultural behavioral changes. Until we have better information concerning variability of salt sensitivity, such a mass attempt at re-education of the public, particularly in view of our other dietary onslaughts on a hopeful but skeptical public, would be ill-advised. Freis suggested editorially that reduction of salt intake to low levels would "wipe out hypertension in several generations,"[22] but his statement at the most is a "provocative suggestion" rather than a pragmatic proposal. Nevertheless, the aforementioned decisions to remove sodium from baby food, and current labeling of food contents are encouraging examples of such cultural progress.

Although we may not easily achieve reduction of sodium intake in normal persons we do have enough data for its use in first-step management of the hypertensive patient. Diminished intake becomes an important part of the nonpharmacological approach to the management of hypertension and is a behaviorally oriented therapy.[23] In addition to being an important first step in the management of the hypertensive, it continues to apply when the patient is then put on a diuretic, since reduction of sodium intake does result in a lesser incidence of the development of hypokalemia from the diuretic.

WEIGHT MANAGEMENT

Obesity is a social and cultural phenomenon which has been clearly demonstrated to play a role in the *predisposition* and *perpetuation* of hypertension. It is not known why the prevalence of hypertension is greater in the obese individual, but much evidence has accumulated that weight reduction does reduce BP. In fact, in our own clinical experience, we find it difficult to effectively lower BP in the hypertensive patient who remains obese. Both epidemiological studies as well as clinical trials have established this relationship, and many of these observations are cited and reviewed by us in Jacob et al.[23] One mechanism that has been suggested for this relationship is that the obese person has perforce an increased sodium intake, but several studies have controlled this factor and shown that weight loss without sodium reduction, does lower BP. Other studies have derived data indicating that drug therapy can be reduced and BP control maintained with weight loss and some have provided data relating actual kilograms of weight lost to mm Hg of BP decline achieved. Examples are the study by Ramsay et al.[24] in which a fall of 2.5/1.5 mm Hg was noted with every Kg of weight decline, and that by Stamler et al.[25] on the Chicago Coronary Prevention Evaluation Program (CPEP) in which 1 Kg of weight loss was associated with a 2.5/1.8 mm Hg decline. Such data give credence to the encouragement we often give our patients that they will lower their BP "1 mm Hg for every pound they lose." In the CPEP study, the weight loss and BP decline were maintained for the 5-year duration of the study in those patients who did not drop out of the program.

Most studies and treatments of obesity in the hypertensive patient have relied on nutrition education interventions, involving the keeping of diaries of food intake along with review of these data and provision of caloric and nutritional advice. Behavioral strategies have been employed to a lesser extent, so that there is a need for their further study and application in the obese hypertensive.

Another aspect of the relationship of obesity to hypertension is the so-called "sleep-apnea syndrome." Unlike the usual "dipping" of BP that occurs during sleep in most hypertensive patients, an undefined number of obese individuals suffer from periods of airway obstruction during sleep which are characterized by marked snoring, apnea, anoxia, and elevation of BP. This syndrome has been associated with an increased incidence of strokes and coronary events in such individuals although the exact prevalence of either the syndrome or its complications is not evident. Nevertheless, relief of the syndrome, by weight loss as well as mechanical nighttime breathing aids and even airway surgery, has been noted to improve hypertension and its control.[26] Further work on this aspect of obesity and it relationship to hypertension, cerebrovascular events, and heart disease is obviously necessary.

OTHER DIETARY INTERVENTIONS

An extensive literature exists of a variety of dietary interventions that have been advocated to treat and/or prevent hypertension. Those that have had perhaps the most interest are potassium intake, calcium intake, and vegetarianism. Reviews of these attempts and outcomes are available, and we will not offer further discussion of them here, except to mention them for the purpose of completeness. Suffice it to say from my own examination of the literature and clinical experience, I do not particularly use any of these modalities in treating my patients. Of particular note is a recent study by Sachs et al.[27] in which significant impact of combinations of potassium, calcium, and magnesium supplements on hypertension control was not apparent.

PHYSICAL EXERCISE

Exercise has been advocated as a method of controlling BP long before it was adopted in the behavioral field. The use of behavioral principles has moved it away from the coaches and fitness experts into the realm of nonpharmacological therapies. Cardiovascular fitness training is of particular pertinence to the management of hypertension. We have reviewed this literature recently[23] and have noted that although aerobic exercise may result in modest reduction of BP in most published studies, significant methodological problems tend to minimize the value of the data. Thus, there is often an absence of no-treatment control groups and the lack of adequate documentation of intermediate variables such as maximal oxygen uptake as a measure of achieved fitness, and the possibility that weight loss is a compounding factor.

The persistence of an exercise effect has been studied by several investigators, who have found a tendency for the lowered levels to increase to baseline levels after discontinuation and a lack of relationship to intensity of the exercise. Conflicting predictors of response have been noted (e.g., low renin values predicted favorable results in one study, whereas high catecholamines were predictive of diminished response in another). Most clinicians warn against the use of isometric exercise in hypertensive patients. Weight lifting, for instance, can cause sharp peaks in BP that are considered potentially dangerous and is ill advised particularly in older individuals, whereas the effects in younger patients have not been impressive.

To summarize, the effects of exercise have not been evaluated with clinical trials methodology. It is likely, however, that small, at least transient, declines can be achieved with improved cardiovascular fitness achieved by aerobic exercise and in our own patients we advocate this lifestyle addition. Most people are increasingly sedentary and when they become aware of the fact that they have an elevated BP, their first reaction is often that they should "take it easy," thus further encouraging inactivity. Patients need to be made aware that exercise is not harmful to their BP, that cardiovascular fitness is improved, that weight loss is helped, and that the exercise need not be of an intense nature. Over the years, we have taken care of many adolescents and young people with modest elevations of BP, who after secondary causes of their hypertension or significant congenital cardiac disease have been ruled out, have participated in often strenuous sports activities, including football, basketball, running, skiing, and so on. without ill effects. To be sure, controlled clinical trials are sparse, and compliance over a long time, as with diet, is a problem in this lifetime disease, but it is a simple nonpharmacological change in lifestyle and we strongly advocate it in patient management, albeit not to the exclusion of pharmacological modalities as needed.

BEHAVIORAL THERAPIES

As mentioned earlier, behavioral methods of treatment have a long history that probably stems from the fact that observers of BP have always noted the variability and reactivity of the pressure under many circumstances, both spontaneously and seemingly induced by whatever is being done to the patient. We have classified the attempts to manipulate BP behaviorally in six categories: psychotherpay, environmental manipulation, placebo, suggestion, biofeedback, and relaxation.

Psychotherapy

Traditional verbal psychotherapy as a method of treating hypertension arose from two concepts. First, because anxiety seemed to elevate BP, its relief by psychotherapy should then lower it. This straightforward relationship requires simple techniques, for example reassurance and supportive psychotherapy. Second, insofar as the hypertensive individual may not be able to handle aggressive and hostile impulses—as suggested by Alexander, Binger, and Dunbar among others—psychodynamic (analytic) therapy might lead to resolution of these conflicts and hence lowering of BP.

Historically, verbal reassurance has played an important role in the management of hypertension. In fact, current attempts at creating public and individual concern about hypertension contrast sharply to attitudes clinicians tried to develop in hypertensive patients before the development of current pharmacologic agents. We reassured patients and discouraged them from worrying about BP levels, based on data that the actual level of BP on any one occasion did not reflect the true status and severity of the ailment or correlate with symptoms; that BP levels were variable and reactive to many stimuli; and that prognosis was often unpredictable and patients might function for many years without disability despite elevated BPs. Patients were not encouraged to take their own BP, ask their physicians its level, or keep personal records of it. The development of a "manometer neurosis" was a matter of concern; reassurance and supportive psychotherapy often with a mild sedative such as phenobarbital, were mainstays of treatment. Environmental manipulation such as job change, rest periods, change of domicile, or domestic arrangements, was frequently recommended. Such treatment, which we have earlier referred to as "a pill and a prayer," was in fact all there was available for the mild and moderate hypertensive, with such therapies as severe sodium restriction and sympathectomy considered as drastic and reserved for patients with severe and progressive disease as defined by end-organ damage rather than BP levels per se.

Two specific studies, one of supportive psychotherapy, the other of analytic therapy, deserve comment in this historical context. The first of these has been alluded to earlier, but is presented here in more detail, namely a study by Reiser et al. done by the Cincinnati group in the early 1950s,[2] before the "pharmacological explosion"; hence this sample of 230 patients received no specific drug therapy. A supportive therapeutic relationship was maintained in 98 of these patients for a minimum of 2 years. Significantly improved BP levels (falls of 20/10 to 40/20 mm Hg) occurred in 22% to 58% of these patients, the degree of impact depending on which of three levels of intensity of supportive psychotherapy they received. Treatment ranged from simple reassurance to superficial insight therapy and was administered by internists, albeit a group with special interest and training in psychosomatic illness. Of further note, 17% to 40% showed improvement in physical findings, whereas 60% reported symptomatic improvement. Of the 98 patients, 17% died, with an average survival of 20 months, but the deaths related to the amount of target-organ damage with which they first presented, rather than to their BP levels. Duration of these salutary effects on BP and other findings was not established in this study. Even at the time, and certainly retrospectively, these outcomes were not impressive in terms of controlling the disease, but they do provide a background that indicates that levels of BP can decline and some improvement ensue without specific therapy and thus at least do speak to the natural history of hypertension.

The second study worthy of comment was that by Moses et al., which was published in 1956,[28] and consisted of only 10 patients, but followed closely in psychoanalytic therapy for up to 6 years. Two of the patients discontinued therapy, but the other 8 showed significant improvement with reduction of pressure to normal (in 4 with mild hypertension) and to a "borderline level" in 2 of the remaining 4. One patient with an accelerated phase of his hypertension, reverted to a benign state with the aid of potent drugs that became available during his course. Moses did not think that as a therapeutic modality, psychoanalysis had a role in the treatment of hypertension per se, being limited by its length, the age and intelligence of the patient, the severity of the psychiatric process, and the degree of reversibility of the somatic state. In the few patients who improved, major reconstructive changes in personality had to be achieved to accomplish the somatic results. There was never any advocacy or enthusiasm about further attempts to utilize psychoanalysis in the treatment of hypertension, but again Moses' work remains as an indication that BP lowering of significance can occur during the course of hypertension, again without specific pharmacologic intervention.

The status of psychotherapy as a therapy for hypertension can thus be summarized from the data described previously, and subsequent reviews, as follows:

1. Declines in blood pressure up to 20 to 40/10 to 30 mm Hg may be achieved and maintained over several years of continued therapy, although subject to "escape" with imposed stress.

2. Patients need to be seen regularly by an experienced therapist, but for supportive therapy it is appropriate and preferable that the therapist be the patient's internist or general physician. For psychoanalytic therapy, an analyst who is "comfortable" with somatic illness is necessary.
3. Supportive therapy is always indicated, especially when drugs are used, because it augments compliance. Any successful provider–patient relationship can offer this basic support.
4. Analytic therapy is highly selective, and the patient's suitability and psychiatric need independent of hypertension determines its use. It is expensive and time consuming.
5. Psychotherapy as treatment clearly has not proceeded beyond a few brief uncontrolled clinical trials, but has a long history of anecdotal experience and pragmatic application.

Environmental Manipulation

Environmental manipulation and modification to lower BP is based on the hypothesis that stressful stimuli arising in a patient's environment adversely affect his or her BP. Considerable epidemiologic evidence that environment influences BP levels is available. Urban populations generally have higher pressures than rural populations. Cultural change, adjustment to a new environment, socioeconomic status, and type of job all have been implicated as affecting BP. Anecdotal examples of improvement with change of environment, job, or home can be provided by most clinicians, and such change is probably recommended to patients frequently without controlled follow-up. However, controlled studies in which change of environment as a therapy has been tested are not available. There are references in the Soviet literature to the use of rest therapy and job adaptation, but with little data.[29]

Data are available concerning certain types of acute changes in environment. For instance, hospitalization generally has a predictable, although variable in degree, effect on BP. In 33 hospitalized hypertensive patients receiving no specific pharmacologic therapy, we reported a maximum fall of *mean* BP of 25.4 ± 19.8 (standard deviation) mm Hg, with this maximum occurring 10 ± 5 days after admission to the hospital.[30] Moutsos and coworkers[31] showed that the placebo effect in six hospitalized patients whose mean BP fell an average of 20 mm Hg was largely the effect of withdrawal from environmental stress. This hospital effect might also relate to the extinction of a conditioned pressor response to BP measurement.

The long-term consequences of hospitalization and other environmental changes are not known. Combining hospitalization with pharmacologic agents is additive and in accelerated hypertension can be an important therapeutic maneuver. Although most patients with benign hypertension can be managed as outpatients, hospitalization is justified when environmental stress causes progressive difficulty in BP control. Hospitalization can have a "negative" effect when conflict between patient and physician or other hospital personnel develops or when problems at home or job are potentiated by the patient's hospitalization.[32] Similarly, any environmental manipulation carries the risk of failing to reduce stress and hence could further exacerbate the BP problem.

To summarize, with the exception of hospitalization, environmental manipulation as a therapy for hypertension primarily has the status of biobehavioral speculation based on epidemiologic data in man and suggestive studies in animal models.[33]

Placebo and Suggestion

The effects of placebos were discussed earlier in regard to their role in evaluating drug therapy. Placebo effects are not treatment modalities but require understanding because they can confound the results achieved by specific therapies, pharmacologic and non-pharmacologic. The *placebo* has been defined as any therapy (or component of therapy) that is used for its nonspecific psychologic and physiologic effect but has no specific pharmacologic impact on the condition being treated.[34] Study of the placebo effect in hypertension has contributed to our knowledge of the phenomenon, but especially it has related to the development of clinical pharmacology and new drug evaluation.[35]

Placebo effects are variable and not always reproducible, the dose-response relations are difficult to identify, and the response is not a necessary consequence of the intent of the treatment. The mechanisms by which the physiologic effects occur are complex and diverse. However, that placebo effects are viewed as nonspecific is a consequence of our current deficiencies in understanding the relations of the multiple factors involved. These factors fall within one of three general categories:[34,36,37]

1. Patient variables—attitudes toward the physician, the treatment, and the illness; levels of anxiety and expectation, education, and past experience with illness.
2. Physician variables—credibility, enthusiasm, authority, empathy, and sympathy.
3. Situational variables—location and form of treatment, interactions with staff and family, content and meaning of instructions and suggestions.

Several conclusions may be drawn from current analyses of placebo effect. First, attempts to define an identifiable "placebo reactive" personality have generally failed.[37,38] Second, placebo effects may adversely affect the clinical course of the patient because side effects, with both subjective and objective symptoms and signs, can be observed with placebo use.[30,38-41] Third, deception is not essential to placebo action, except in the special case of "blind" drug trials. Fourth, the doctor (provider)–patient relationship is the agency of the placebo effect.[42]

Magnitude of Placebo and Suggestion Effects on BP. Placebo factors include various psychological influences and manipulations that may be associated with systematic directional shifts in BP.[2,30,43,44] BP changes in most studies are in the same range of magnitude as those described with procedures discussed elsewhere in this chapter (about 5 to 25 mm Hg, systolic or diastolic).

The salutary effect of a sustained therapeutic relation in the hypertensive patient was mentioned earlier. The converse effect, an adverse response to a negative change in the physician's attitudes and enthusiasm—which partially negated the effect of both the placebo and the antihypertensive drug under study,[39] despite a double-blind experimental design—also has been described. Wolf and colleagues[44] and Pickering[46] likewise have noted a potent role for the doctor–patient relationship as an adjunct or deterrent to pharmacotherapy.

Certain variables that cannot be easily separated from placebo effects are relevant to the procedures described here. The first appearance of a patient at treatment site often has a pressor effect, probably related to apprehension. Accommodation to the situation results in a relative decline in BP, appearing to be improvement. The use of placebo as an "antihypertensive" medication may or may not result in lower BP; this outcome depends on physician attitudes, severity of hypertension, and whether comparison is made with initial visits, nontreatment periods, or hospitalization.[46-49,59]

An older but classic study of suggestion in 1955 by Goldring and associates[50] of 31 outpatients shows the effect of intensive reassurance combined with visual exposure to a dramatic but innocuous device, which subjects were informed was a "therapeutic electron gun." BPs fell an average of 20/14 mm Hg; in eight of the patients DBP fell below 90 mm Hg, an average diastolic fall of 25 mm Hg. Although the effect lasted only several weeks and a precise experimental design was lacking, these data have special pertinence to biofeedback, relaxation, and psychotherapy studies. Similarly, numerous stimuli may result in acute BP elevations in normotensive and hypertensive persons, for example, stressful interviews,[44] the amount of interpersonal interaction,[51] forced perception of conflict,[52] psychodrama involving assertiveness or hostility,[53] and frustrating or demanding verbal and mental tasks.[54,55] Removal of the noxious stimulus in these situations results in a return of pressures to baseline that might be interpreted as resulting from a specific therapeutic intervention.

Suggestion as a therapeutic factor also has been shown in experiments involving direct verbal instruction to control BP without biofeedback or meditation with appropriate directional changes of 15/10 mm Hg.[45,56] In some studies of voluntary control of BP, instruction appears crucial to responses,[48,57-58] and in most studies involving hypertensive persons, awareness of the task required—that is, to lower BP—occurs either explicitly or is surmised by the patient. Such awareness of therapeutic intent clearly influences the response to medications[60,61] and will facilitate voluntary control of other autonomic responses[62,63] posing a further problem in evaluating the specificity of behavioral therapies.

Evaluation of Placebo Effects. Placebo influences produce a summation of social, attitudinal, and environmental factors that affect the BP levels of hypertensive patients. Awareness of these factors has led to the design of elaborate control procedures for evaluating antihypertensive drugs, and such procedures are equally necessary for the rational assessment of nonpharmacologic therapies. Although the placebo effect is potent, it is not proposed as a planned therapeutic approach to the management of hypertension in the present era of pharmacological and nonpharmacological therapies, but its impact on the patient and on evaluation of therapy must be continually recognized. Similarly, suggestion per se will influence outcome although again it has little if any lasting value.

Biofeedback

As stated by Miller,[64] *biofeedback* is the

> use of modern instrumentation to give better moment-to-moment information about a specific physiologic process that is under the control of the nervous system but not clearly or accurately perceived. In the terminology of "servo systems," such information has been called feedback. Such information about a biologic process is called biofeedback. (p. 684)

With the aid of this information, one may develop some control over a physiologic process.

Historically, responses innervated by the ANS were considered "involuntary" and not modified by trial-and-error learning (also termed *instrumental* or *operant conditioning*). However, it is now documented that when animals or humans are provided with feedback for different physiologic processes and are given appropriate incentives for controlling the responses, they can learn to self-regulate functions such as HR, BP, blood flow, skin temperature, sweat gland activity, and gastric and intestinal processes.[65,66]

Neither the peripheral nor central mechanisms involved in the self-regulation of BP are clearly known. Changes in muscle tension and respiration may be contributing factors but are not the sole mechanisms. Differential control of HR and BP can be achieved, depending on the specific type of biofeedback. For instance, in studies by Schwartz[67] and D. Shapiro and coworkers,[68-70] normotensive subjects learned to change *either* HR or SBP, or both simultaneously, and in *either* direction, with different kinds of biofeedback aimed at the patterns in which these different physiologic changes were recurring. Importantly, simultaneous changes in BP and HR also may occur if subjects are given specific instructions to control these functions, and they then will draw on various cognitive and somatic strategies to produce more complex physiologic patterns. Because BP is the outcome of the relation between cardiac output and peripheral resistance, then depending on the type of biofeedback and instructions used, changes in HR, stroke volume, and peripheral resistance may be differentially involved, the exact details of each needing specification. In addition, biofeedback for other potentially relevant physiologic responses, such as muscle tension (electromyography), sweat gland activity (galvanic skin response), and skin temperature theoretically may aid in lowering BP.[71,72]

Biofeedback methods use diverse techniques. Most effective are constant pressure cuff systems with which binary (yes–no) feedback for increase or decrease of BP at each beat can be given. The system is usually more reliable for SBP than for DBP. More intermittent biofeedback procedures based on a standard cuff system obviously cannot be used to recognize rapid changes in BP but may aid patients to self-monitor or regulate pressure both in the laboratory and at home. Ambulatory indirect monitors can be adapted for such use. Various types of "rewards" are used for lowering BP or achieving objectives, but praise and support from family and therapist along with the patient's desire for self-regulation are major incentives in the process. The magnitude of BP decline with biofeedback has been reviewed in numerous publications, and has not appreciably changed from what we described in a review of the then existing data in 1977;[73] it is usually modest and generally does not exceed approximately 20/10 mm Hg. How permanent such effects are and their value in the long term for chronic hypertension is discussed in more detail in the subsequent section on relaxation therapies.

Relaxation Therapy

Relaxation therapy is a form of stress management and has a long history. Practitioners of certain Eastern disciplines and religions, notably Zen and Yoga, for hundreds of years have reported the ability to control autonomically regulated functions. Consideration of biofeedback methods in the treatment of hypertension reawakened interest in these older methods of relaxation and led to a number of new and perhaps simpler techniques. As with biofeedback, the revision of traditional opinion that the ANS is beyond conscious control encouraged this progress.

Relaxation methods, although differing in specifics and focus, seek to elicit calmness and a hypometabolic state. The response is associated with decreased sympathetic arousal and heightened activity in the supraoptic and preoptic areas of the anterior hypothalamus.[74,75] This integrated state of lowered sympathetic activity might be expected to lower BP, because essential hypertensive subjects show a reactive pressor response to stimuli and the sympathetic nervous system is the major mediator of this response.[76-78]

Several specific relaxation methods have been proposed for the treatment of hypertension. They have been reviewed in several publications[73,78] and are summarized here:

1. Progressive relaxation (Jacobsonian): a technique directed at relaxation of major skeletal muscle groups.
2. Autogenic training: standard "autosuggestive" exercises for inducing altered physiologic and mental states.
3. Hypnotic relaxation: hypnosis and posthypnotic suggestion to induce physiologic and mental relaxation.
4. Zen meditation: methods of meditation involving passive concentration on respiration and a logical exercise (koans) to elicit the relaxation response.

5. Hatha yoga: relaxation is elicited through bodily postures and exercises (asanas), breath control (pranayana), and meditation (dhyana).
6. Transcendental meditation: a cognitive technique derived from Vedic practices in which individuals assume a comfortable position, breath peacefully, close the eyes, and repeat a "mantra" (a Sanskrit word or sound) as each breath is exhaled.
7. Relaxation response: a simplified and standardized meditative technique developed by Benson and coworkers based on transcendental meditation and Zen and specifically directed to relaxation, but tailored more to Western culture.

None of these methods were specifically devised for treatment of hypertension. All claim nonspecific benefits for lifestyle and "well-being," as well as their potential for hypotensive effects. The abbreviated descriptions fail to do justice to the emphasis and contextual variables that give each method its particular character. Benefits from each technique are enhanced by a trained clinician or teacher, who initiates and instructs the patient, gives encouragement and corrective feedback, and follows progress and compliance.

The magnitude of effects with relaxation and stress management techniques are modest and increasingly less impressive. Following the initial enthusiasm for their use, the effects have been shown to be relatively transient and not particularly evident outside of the laboratory, as for instance when ambulatory, day-long monitoring is performed. Effects on endpoints other than BP have not been achieved, with the possible exception of studies by Patel[80,81] who showed effects lasting up to 12 months associated with decrease in drug requirements and in a few patients a decline in morbidity, but her studies have not been repeated or confirmed by other investigators. An interesting observation by Stone and deLeo[82] did show some decline in plasma renin activity and components of the catecholamine system that were cited as evidence of decrease in adrenergic activity along with BP, but whether cause or effect remains unanswered. Relaxation effects are also not easily distinguished from those due to sleep, particularly because some studies show EEG patterns of sleep during transcendental meditation, for instance. Recent studies by Chesney et al.[83] and Agras et al.[84] have been discouraging in terms of the specificity of relaxation as a therapeutic modality in that they failed to show a long-term advantage of behavioral therapy over BP monitoring in the research clinic. In both trials, there was a progressive decline in BP in the control groups during monitoring in the clinic or work site. These studies emphasize the need to monitor for a period of time, before adding relaxation, a fact that has been well known to the clinical pharmacologist evaluating drugs.

We recently summarized our concerns and doubts about the specificity of relaxation and other behavioral therapies in a review questioning whether the effects of stress management really represent just regression to the mean and related factors.[59] As results of better designed studies have accumulated, the clinical effects appear less convincing. Larger BP declines tend to be reported in studies that do not include adequate baseline assessments. Habituation to a new environment, as may occur in a subject attending a new clinic, treatment program, or provider plays a role in eliciting BP decline as does the development of a therapeutic relationship with the physician or other provider. Differential effects in habituation between control and treatment groups may occur as related to waiting periods before therapy is started. Drop-out rates may differ; in some studies, drop-out rates are higher in the behavioral treatment patients than in controls or even in drug studies. Certainly, compliance is a major problem in behavioral studies, particularly when such treatments require home practice by the patient. Carryover effects into the environment are also questionable. In a study of our own comparing drugs and relaxation with measurements done at different sites, the most favorable results were seen on BP changes within a relaxation session; conversely, no relaxation effect was noted on automated ambulatory monitoring outside of the therapist's laboratory or in the hypertension clinic when seen by the patient's usual physician.[85]

These findings are consistent with the notion that relaxation produces a state opposite to that of "stress." In effect, whereas stress produces a transient pressor response, relaxation induces a transient depressor response. The situational specificity of the relaxation effect suggests that it is similar to the placebo response.[86] In a recent study by Gould et al. using intra-arterial ambulatory monitoring, it was observed that the placebo effect was limited to the clinic setting, while active drug effects were also observed in other environments.[87] I am not aware of any studies on relaxation therapy that have noted significant declines during ambulatory monitoring.

Self-quieting maneuvers may be acquired by subjects in any therapeutic study and are particularly pertinent in evaluating outcomes in behavioral studies. Thus, patients may "learn" quickly to "sit still" when BP is being measured and this ability may be different between treated and control groups.

Summary of Outcomes of Behavioral Therapies

Over the many years of our clinical and research involvement with the management of hypertension, we have given much thought to the use of behavioral techniques, and practiced most of them at one time or another. In fact, as we have repeatedly mentioned, such methods were all that were available in the "early days." Certain usages, such as reassurance and resistance to panic—both on the part of the patient as well as the doctor—when finding an unusually high pressure, have remained a part of my therapeutic armamentarium in the present era of specific and effective drug therapy. My interests in biofeedback and relaxation treatments were primarily research-oriented and I believe that from our own work and from review of the contributions of many others, we have come to certain conclusions. Relaxation and biofeedback have provided us with further evidence of the reactivity and variability of BP in the hypertensive patient. Just as stress studies have clearly delineated the pressor response as a feature of BP control, which may cause detrimental consequences in the predisposition, precipitation, and perpetuation of hypertensive disease, the behavioral therapies have established the existence of a depressor response, which may in the short-term occasionally have ameliorative consequences, at least on BP alone. As such, the lowering of BP by relaxation is an epiphenomenon. It is the converse of the well-established pressor response, involving varied depressor mechanisms—ANS, hormonal, and local—of considerable interest in understanding BP control, but of minimal clinical significance in the long-term management of hypertension. Similar conclusions regarding the effectiveness of cognitive behavioral therapies have been reached in a recent meta-analysis reported by Eisenberg et al.[88]

REFERENCES

1. Reiser MF, Rosenbaum M, Ferris EB. Psychologic mechanisms in malignant hypertension. *Psychosom Med.* 1951;13:147-159.
2. Reiser MF, Brust AA, Shapiro AP, Baker HM, Ransohoff W, Ferris EB. Life situations, emotions and the course of patients with arterial hypertension. *Psychosom Med.* 1951;13:133-139.
3. Veteran's Administration Cooperative Study Group on Antihypertensive Agents, I. Results in patients with diastolic blood pressures of 115 through 129 mm Hg. *JAMA.* 1967;202:1028-1034.
4. Veteran's Administration Cooperative Study Group on Antihypertensive Agents. II. Effects of treatment on morbidity in hypertension: Results in patients with diastolic blood pressures averaging 90 through 114 mm Hg. *JAMA.* 1970;213:1143-1152.
5. Veteran's Administration Cooperative Study Group on Antihypertensive Agents. III. Influence of age, diastolic pressure, and prior cardiovascular disease: Further analysis of side effects. *Circ.* 1972;45:991-1004.
6. Five year findings of the Hypertension Detection and Followup Program. I. Reduction in mortality of persons with high blood pressure, including mild hypertension. HDFP Cooperative Group, DHEW: (AP Shapiro, Chairman, Policy Advisory Board) *JAMA.* 1979; 242:2562-2571.
7. Five year findings of the Hypertension Detection and Followup Program. II. Mortality by race, sex and age. HDFP cooperative Group, DHEW: (A.P. Shapiro, Chairman, Policy Advisory Board) *JAMA.* 1979;242:2572-2577.
8. Denton DA. Evolutionary aspects of the emergence of aldosterone secretion and salt appetite. *Physiol Rev.* 1965;45:245-293.
9. Cassel J. Hypertension and cardiovascular disease in migrants: a potential source of clues. *Int J Epidemiol.* 1974;3:204-206.
10. Henry JP. Stress, salt, and hypertension. *Social Sci and Med.* 1988;26:293-302.
11. Page LB, Damon A, Moellering RC. Antecedents of cardiovascular disease in six Solomon Island societies. *Circ.* 1974;49:2232 2246.
12. Oliver WJ, Cohen EL, Neal JV. Blood pressure, sodium intake, and sodium related hormones in the Yanomano Indians. *Circ.*1975; 52:146-151.
13. Wilson TW, Grim CE. Biohistory of slavery and blood pressure differences in blacks today: an hypothesis. *Hypertension.* 1991;17(suppl. I):I122-I128.
14. Parijs J, Joossens JV, Van der Linden L, Verstreken G, Amery AKPC. Moderate sodium restriction and diuretics in the treatment of hypertension. *Am Heart J.* 1973;85:22-34.
15. Morgan T, Adam W, Gillies A, Wilson M, Morgan G, Carney S. Hypertension treated by salt restriction. *Lancet.* 1978;1:227-230.
16. Singer DRJ, Markandu ND, Capuccio FP, Miller MA, Sagnella GA, MacGregor GA. Reduction of salt intake during converting enzyme inhibitor treatment compared with addition of a thiazide. *Hypertension.* 1995; 25:1042-1044.
17. Luft F, Bloch R, Weyman A, Murray A, Weinberger M. Cardiovascular responses to extremes of salt intake in man. *Clin Res.* 1978;26:365A.
18. Menely GR, Ball COT. Experimental epidemiology of chronic sodium chloride toxicity and the protective effect of potassium chloride. *Am J Med.* 1958;25:713-725.

19. Dahl LK. Effects of chronic excess salt feeding: induction of self-sustaining hypertension in rats. *J Exp Med.* 1961;114:231-236.
20. Kawasaki T, Delea CS, Bartter FC, Smith H. The effect of high sodium and low sodium intakes on blood pressure and other related variables in human subjects with idiopathic hypertension. *Am J Med.* 1978;64:293-298.
21. Langford HG, Watson RL, Thomas JG. Salt intake and the treatment of hypertension. *Am Heart J.* 1977;93:531-532.
22. Freis ED. Salt, volume and the prevention of hypertension. *Circ.* 1976;53:589-595.
23. Jacob RG, Wing R, Shapiro AP. The behavioral treatment of hypertension: Long-term effects. *Behavior Therapy.* 1987;18:325-352.
24. Ramsay LE, Ramsay MH, Hettiaracchi J, Davies DL, Winchester J. Weight reduction in a blood pressure clinic. *Brit Med J.* 1978;2:244-245.
25. Stamler J, Farinaro E, Mojonnier LM, Hall Y, Moss D, Stamler R. Prevention and control of hypertension by nutritional-hygienic means. *JAMA.* 1980;243:1819-1823.
26. Fletcher FC. The relationship between systemic hypertension and obstructive sleep apnea: facts and theory. *Am J Med.* 1995;98:118-128.
27. Sachs FM, Brown LE, Appel L, Borhani NO, Evans D, Whelton P. Combination of potassium, calcium, and magnesium supplements in hypertension. *Hypertension.* 1995;26:950-956.
28. Moses L, Daniels GE, Nickerson JL. Psychogenic factors in essential hypertension. *Psychosom Med.* 1956;18:471-485.
29. Simonson E, Brozek J. Russian research in arterial hypertension. *Ann Intern Med.* 1959;50:129-193.
30. Shapiro AP. Consideration of the multiple variables involved in the evaluation of hypotensive agents. *JAMA.* 1956;160:30-39.
31. Moutsos SE, Sapira JD, Scheib ET, Shapiro AP. An analysis of the placebo effect in hospitalized hypertensive patients. *Clin Pharmacol Ther.* 1967;8:676-683.
32. Shapiro AP. Cardiovascular disorders. In: Waife SO, Shapiro AP, eds. Clinical Evaluation of New Drugs. New York: Hoeber-Harper; 1959:135-152.
33. Henry JP, Cassel JC. Psychosocial factors in essential hypertension: epidemiologic and animal experimental evidence. *Am J Epidemiol.* 1969;90:171 180.
34. Shapiro AK. Semantics of the placebo. *Psychiatr Q.* 1968;42:653-695.
35. Smith WM, Melmon KL. Drug choice in disease. In: Melman KL, Morelli HF, eds. *Clinical Pharmacology.* New York: Macmillan; 1972:3-20.
36. Liberman R. An analysis of the placebo phenomena. *J Chronic Dis.* 1962;15:761-783.
37. Shapiro AK. Placebo effects in medicine, psychotherapy, and psychoanalysis. In: Bergin AE, Garfield, SL, eds. *Handbook on Pyschotherapy and Behavioral Change.* New York: Aldine; 1971:439-473.
38. Beecher HK. Placebos and the evaluation of the subjective response. In: Waife SO, Shapiro AP, eds. *The Clinical Evaluation of New Drugs.* New York: Hoeber-Harper; 1959:62-75.
39. Shapiro AP, Myers T, Reiser MF, Ferris EB. Comparison of blood pressure response to veriloid with that to the doctor-patient relationship. *Psychosom Med.* 1954;15:478-488.
40. Uhlenhuth EH, Cantor A, Neustadt JD, et al. The sympatomatic relief of anxiety with meprobamate, phenobarbital and placebo. *Am J Psychiatry.* 1959;115:905-910.
41. Wolf S. The pharmacology of placebos. *Pharmacol Rev.* 1959;11:629-704.
42. Adler HM, Hammett VO. The doctor-patient relationship revisited. An analysis of the placebo effect. *Ann Intern Med.* 1973;78:595-598.
43. Alexander F. Emotional factors in essential hypertension. *Psychosom Med.* 1939;1:173-179.
44. Wolf S, Cardon PV, Shepard EM, et al. Life stress and essential hypertension. a study of circulatory adjustments in man. Baltimore: Williams & Wilkins, 1955.
45. Shapiro AP, Redmond DP, McDonald RH Jr, Gaylor M. Relationships of perception, cognition, suggestion and operant conditioning in essential hypertension. In: Gispen WH, Van Wimersma Greidanus TJB, Bohus B, De Wied D. *Hormones, Homeostasis and the Brian: Progress in Brain Research.* Amsterdam: Elsevier Scientific Publishing Co; 1975:299-312.

46. Pickering, G.W. *High blood pressure.* 2nd ed. London: Churchill; 1968.
47. Freis ED (Chairman). VAH cooperative study group: a double blind control study of anti-hypertensive agents. *Arch Intern Med.* 1960;106:133-148.
48. Shapiro D, Schwartz GE, Tursky B. Control of diastolic blood pressure in man by feedback and reinforcement. *Psychophysiol.* 1972;9:296-304.
49. Shapiro AP, Teng HC. Technique of controlled drug assay illustrated by a comparative study of Rauwolfia serpentina, phenobarbital, and placebo in the hypertensive patient. *NEJM.* 1957;256:970-995.
50. Goldring W, Chasis H, Schreiner GF, et al. Reassurance in the management of benign hypertensive disease. *Circ.* 1956; 14:260-264.
51. Williams RB, Kimball CP, Williard HN. The influence of interpersonal interaction in diastolic blood pressure. *Psychosom Med.* 1972;34:194-198.
52. Sapira JD, Scheib ET, Moriarty R, Shapiro AP. Difference in perception between hypertensive and normotensive populations. *Psychosom Med.* 1971;33:239-250.
53. Kalis BL, Harris RE, Sokolow M. Response to psychological stress in patients with essential hypertension. *Am Heart J.* 1957;53:572-578.
54. Brod J, Fencl V, Hejl Z, Jirka J. Circulatory changes underlying blood pressure elevation during acute emotional stress. *Clin Sci.* 1959;18:269-279.
55. Shapiro AP. An experimental study of comparative responses of blood pressure to noxious stimuli. *J Chronic Dis.* 1961;13:293-311.
56. Redmond DP, Gaylor MS, McDonald RH Jr, Shapiro AP. Blood pressure and heart rate response to verbal instructions and relaxation in hypertension. *Psychosom Med.* 1974;36:285.
57. Brener J, Kleinman RA. Learned control of decreases in systolic blood pressure. *Nature.* 1970;226:1063-1064.
58. Brener J. A general model of voluntary control applied to the phenomena of learned cardiovascular change. In: Obrist PA, Black AH, Brener J, eds. *Cardiovascular Psychophysiology.* Chicago: Aldine; 1974:365-391.
59. Jacob RG, Shapiro AP. Is the effect of stress management on blood pressure just regression to the mean? *Hemeostatis.* 1994;35:113-119.
60. Knowles JB, Lucas CJ. Experimental studies of the placebo response. *J Ment Sci.* 1960;106:231-240.
61. Sternbach RA. The effects of instructional sets on autonomic responsivity. *Psychophysiol.* 1964;1:67-72.
62. Bergman JS, Johnson HJ. Sources of information which affect training and raising of heart rate. *Psychophysiol.* 1972;9:30-39.
63. Blanchard EB, Scott RW, Young ID, et al. Effect of knowledge of response on the self-control of heart rate. *Psychophysiol.* 1974;11:251-264.
64. Miller NE. Biofeedback; evaluation of a new technique (editorial). *NEJM.* 1974;290:684-685.
65. Miller NE. Learning of visceral and glandular responses. *Science.* 1969;163:434-445.
66. Shapiro D, Schwartz GE. Biofeedback and visceral learning: Clinical applications. *Semin Psychiatry.* 1972;4:171-184.
67. Schwartz GE. Toward a theory of voluntary control of response patterns in the cardiovascular system. In: Obrist PA, Black AH, Brener, J, eds. *Cardiovascular Psychophysiology.* Chicago: Aldine; 1974:406-441.
68. Shapiro D, Tursky B, Gershown E, et al. Effects of feedback and reinforcement on the control of human systolic blood pressure. *Science.* 1969;163:588-589.
69. Shapiro D, Tursky B, Schwartz GE. Control of blood pressure in man by operant conditioning. *Circ Res.* 1970;26(suppl 1):1-27-1-32.
70. Shapiro D, Tursky B, Schwartz GE. Differentiation of heart rate and blood pressure in man by operant conditioning. *Psychosom Med.* 1970;32:417-423.
71. Schwartz GE. Biofeedback as therapy: some theoretical and practical issues. *Am Psychol.* 1973;28:666-673.

72. Shapiro D, Mainardi JA, Surwit RS. Biofeedback and self-regulation in essential hypertension. In: Schwartz GE, Beatty J, eds. *Biofeedback: Theory and Research.* New York: Academic Press; 1976.
73. Shapiro AP, Schwartz GE, Ferguson DCE, Redmond DP, Weiss SM. Behavioral methods in the treatment of hypertension. *Ann Intern Med.* 1977;86:626-636.
74. Hess WR. *Functional organization of the diencephalon.* New York: Grune & Stratton; 1957.
75. Beary JF, Benson H, Klemchuk HP. A simple physiologic technique which elicits the hypometabolic changes of the relaxation response. *Psychosom Med.* 1974;36:115-120.
76. Benson H. *The relaxation response.* New York: William Morrow; 1975.
77. Benson H, Beary JF, Carol MP. The relaxation response. *Psychiatry.* 1974;37:37-46.
78. Abboud FM. Relaxation, autonomic control, and hypertension (editorial). *NEJM.* 1976;294:107-109.
79. Schwartz GE, Shapiro AP, Redmond DP, Ferguson DCE, Ragland DR, Weiss SM. Behavioral medicine approaches to hypertension: an integrative analysis of theory and research. *J Behav Med.* 1979;2:311-363.
80. Patel CH. Twelve-month follow-up of yoga and biofeedback in the management of hypertension. *Lancet.* 1975;1:62-64.
81. Patel CH, North WR. Randomized control trial of yoga and biofeedback in management of hypertension. *Lancet.* 1975;2:93-95.
82. Stone RA, DeLeo J. Psychotherapeutic control of hypertension. *NEJM.* 1976;294:80-84.
83. Chesney MA, Black GW, Swan GE, Ward MM. Relaxation training for essential hypertension at the Worksite I. The untreated hypertensive. *Psychosom Med.* 1987;49:250-263.
84. Agras WS, Taylor CB, Kraemer HC, Southam MA, Schneider JA. Relaxation training for essential hypertension at the worksite: II. The poorly controlled hypertensive. *Psychosom Med.* 1987;49:264-273.
85. Jacob RG, Shapiro AP, O'Hara P, Portser S, Kruger A, Gatsonis C, Ding Y. Relaxation therapy for hypertension: setting specific effects. *Psychosom Med.* 1992;54:87-101.
86. Jacob RG, Shapiro AP, Reeves RA, Johnsen AM, McDonald RH Jr, Coburn PC. Relaxation therapy for hypertension. Comparison of effects with concomitant placebo, diuretic, and betablocker. *Arch Intern Med.* 1986;146:2335-2340.
87. Gould BP, Mann S, Davies AB, Altman DG, Raferty EB. Does placebo lower blood pressure? *Health Psychol.* 1987;6:399-416.
88. Eisenberg DM, Delbanco TL, Berkey CS, Kaptchuk TJ, Kupelnick B, Kuhl J, Chalmers TC. Cognitive behavioral techniques for hypertension: are they effective? *Ann Int Med.* 1993;118:964-972.

7

Compliance With Therapy

As physicians, we often assume in our omniscience that what we tell our patients to do, is done. We write our magical prescriptions that are then carefully filled by our colleagues, the pharmacists, and we expect our patients to administer our potions regularly and consistently. If therapeutic results are achieved, we congratulate ourselves that we have fulfilled our contract; if the therapy fails we blame it on noneffectiveness of the particular treatment, the intractibility of the ailment, or—with occasional humility—on our mistaken diagnosis. That the patient is not taking the medication or conforming to the behavior that we prescribed when results are not forthcoming is a consideration to which we usually do not give primary attention. Yet compliance with our recommendations is a major factor in our success, and noncompliance, advertently or inadvertently, severely diminishes our efforts. Even when outcomes are as we would predict and the patient is doing well, we may delude ourselves into assuming that compliance is practiced, when in fact we are only observing the natural history of the disease or regression to the mean. These considerations are particularly pertinent when dealing with the treatment of hypertension, when—for reasons we have discussed earlier and repeatedly—the measurement we use, BP, is so variable.

The evaluation and study of compliance with therapy is of course a universal consideration with any therapy. However, it is a particular need in the management of hypertensive disease because it is a chronic ailment. The mind set in most diseases is that if one is ill or feels poorly, medication is taken for a period of time until the symptoms and signs have abated and then the treatment is discontinued. With hypertension, in contrast, one usually feels well when treatment is started and may indeed trade this feeling of well-being for a symptomatic state related to the medication, or at best continue to be asymptomatic relying for satisfaction only on the rewards of being told that "your BP is better." Moreover, the medication must be continued for an undefined lengthy period, often for a lifetime, and usually in an outpatient setting in which the patient is otherwise living a normal life and taking part in his or her usual daily activities. Accordingly, management of hypertension has become a leading arena for the study of compliance.[1] Control of hypertension and diminution of morbidity and mortality from the disease, as has been demonstrated in large-scale clinical trials as well as in smaller individual studies and epidemiological data collections, are predicated on the assumption that patients will comply with recommended therapy; it thus behooves us to recognize the predominant importance of this parameter of treatment. Moreover, the psychological and social factors that influence compliance make its evaluation truly an endeavor that requires study of human behavior.

Many factors interfere with compliance. The consensus from a number of studies indicates that as many as one third of patients fail to adhere to prescribed therapy. As mentioned earlier, belief in an acute disease model for hypertension rather than the chronic disease model is a major cause of loss of compliance. Side effects from medication, either actual, feared, or perceived, cause many patients to stray from their prescribed routines. In my own practice, mostly now as a consultant for difficult to manage patients, the most frequent problem with which I am faced is the patient who complains that he or she has received many different drugs and "all of them" cause problems. Some of the problems are easily understood because they represent unwanted but predictable or expected pharmacological consequences of the drug in question, but often the complaints are not traceable to any property of the agent in question and may be rather nonspecific or even bizarre. In some patients, one almost gets the impression of virtually a conditioned reflex wherein any medication taken causes distress. One finds it difficult, for instance, to ascribe a feeling of numbness in one hand occurring within minutes of taking a diuretic drug orally to any known pharmacologic action of that drug, and yet such complaints have been expressed by certain of my patients. To the patient this is a real problem; no amount of reassurance or denial of the connection by the provider can persuade the patient differently, and the result is noncompliance at least with that particular drug. The most that the physician can accomplish in such instances is to preserve the doctor–patient relationship sufficiently to get the patient to try something else.

The cost of the medication is clearly a source of noncompliance and it is not simply the issue of the hypertensive mother of several small children who must choose between her medication and new shoes for her child. It may equally be the problem of the husband who will willingly pay several dollars a day for his cigarettes and liquor and resent spending a usually lesser amount for his daily medication. Somehow in his thinking, he is "entitled" to the former, whereas the latter is an imposition that furthermore impacts his manly image. The problem is not abrogated by providing the medication and the clinic visits at little or no cost; in our study in a Veterans Hospital setting where care cost to the patient is minimal to nonexistent, the one third noncompliance rate was still present. Of interest in these studies was the fact that compliance was poorer in younger patients rather than in the older.[2] This observation is compatible with the probability that noncompliance can also be a product of denial, to wit, the young conceive themselves to be healthy and even immortal, in contrast to older folk who are increasingly realizing the inevitability of their need for medical care. Hence, the theme "Hypertension—the Silent Killer" has been used now for several decades as a major threat in education programs about the need for detection and treatment.

The frequency of the administration of the medication during the course of the day is a much studied component of compliance. As might be expected, a drug given once a day achieves better compliance than one requiring multiple administrations. Twice a day is almost as effective as once a day and can be associated by the patient with another specific daily activity, whereas administrations beyond that number become increasingly difficult to remember. Forgetfulness is obviously a frequent cause of noncompliance, particularly in the older patient in whom loss of memory is now a disease and not merely a lapse of awareness. Education in associative techniques (e.g., "take your pills in the morning [and/or evening] right after you've brushed your teeth") is the simplest way to handle this problem of remembering. Social support from the "nagging spouse" who lays out the daily ration of pills for the patient is also a solution, but can be counterproductive and can fail to encourage the need for the patient to become him or herself responsible.

The lifestyle and working habits of the patient can interfere with compliance; for example, the patient who works (or plays) on a varying schedule, or travels and cannot (or forgets to) carry his or her pills has an obvious problem. It is often necessary to supply the patient with a written list of what he or she is taking and the schedule for administration. More compulsive patients will prepare their own list, whereas the compulsive physician or provider will prepare it for them and review it at each visit. The prescription labeling by the pharmacist may be insufficient, particularly when medication changes are often made both in dose and type of medication or the patient "for convenience" removes the pill from its original vial and puts it in another container. It is also wise as part of patient education in compliance to teach the patient the names of the drugs being taken, as well as their dose size, the latter sometimes requiring basic instruction in the metric system because in the United States most people still have not been taught to think in metrics and drug doses are now all compounded by that system.

Level of education in general influences compliance, but there are notable exceptions as with the "overeducated" and seemingly medically sophisticated patient who may try to "outguess" the provider by making changes on his or her own. This has been a particular problem in recent years when new medical "breakthroughs" or dire information about particular drugs are trumpeted in the popular press before legitimate publications have reached the desk of even the well-informed physician. A barrage of phone calls after such releases can be expected either frantically wondering about continuing to comply with prescribed medications or demanding information on new ones, which must be handled with patience and tact if effective compliance is to be maintained.

Gender is a factor in compliance. Several studies have indicated that men are more apt to be noncompliant than women and that young men are especially difficult to keep in therapy. This may have to do with the male "macho image" to which we have previously alluded, particularly because male impotence is frequently attributed to various of the medications used in treating hypertension. Although often without a pharmacological reason for this sexual failure, it is nevertheless a common belief by many men; with their usual sensitivity about impotence, it is difficult to persuade such patients otherwise and usually medication changes should and must be made to maintain compliance at least with some type therapy.

Compliance also varies depending on the demographics of study. For instance, some studies have shown that patients in a family practice setting have better rates of compliance, while those in an HMO setting and in hospital clinics had the poorer rates whereas counseling by nurses and other nonphysician providers, improved compliance. However, in the excellent review of compliance problems by Dunbar-Jacob et al.,[3] to which we are indebted for much of the information in our current discussion, it is pointed out that the variations noted in the different settings described here cannot be as yet cited as reasons to devise new strategies for hypertension health care delivery. Other variations in delivery such as patient characteristics have not been thoroughly accounted for in these studies that also were not designed experimentally but are essentially descriptive. Nevertheless, from our experiences in several large-scale clinical trials such as the HDFP and MRFIT, in which compliance was excellent, it would certainly appear that intensive special care with compulsive pursuit of the patients' attendance, counseling, education, and so on are productive.

It is worth noting, in view of the argument that pharmacological drop-out and compliance rates are such that nonpharmacological treatments should be pursued as alternatives, that reported data have not confirmed this hypothesis. Dunbar-Jacob et al. in their review of compliance studies in the last decade, indicated a relaxation study with only a 39% compliance rate with drug study rates of 38% to 95% in a series of varied studies. Admittedly, motivation plays a role in such comparisons; for instance in our experience when relaxation techniques were employed in patients coming to a hypertension clinic for pharmacological therapy who were asked to enter a relaxation study, refusals and drop-outs were high, whereas among patients directly volunteering for such nonpharmacological therapies much better compliance was maintained. Similarly, compliance with weight reduction and sodium restricting programs are as difficult to maintain as drug studies, and in fact many of our patients will readily point out that they would rather "take a pill regularly" than struggle with dietary restrictions.

Techniques for studies of compliance have been thoroughly examined in the review by Dunbar-Jacob et al. The standard methods used by most investigators are self-reports and pill counts; both have effectiveness and show modest correlations with each other. Similarly, their correlations with BP control are modest but some are statistically significant. The problems with both of these methods are obvious; patients motivated to "fool" the investigators are easily able to conceal their actual behaviors. Pharmacy records have also been used but again are only valid when the pharmacy being used is the only one that the patient has available and it is assumed that any pills obtained are used and pills not obtained are not used. Only a few studies have looked at biological indices, at least one with propranolol levels and several others with either thiazide blood or urine levels. Such studies are quite expensive and although they will correlate with self-reports of compliance, and actually probably be more reliable, it is not clear that they correlate with BP outcomes any better than the subjective techniques.

A reliable measure of compliance, however, should not have to correlate with BP outcome in order to demonstrate its validity. It is quite possible of course that a fully compliant patient has poor BP lowering with a given drug even though he or she is taking the medication faithfully; our goal is to establish that the failure of BP to respond is not caused by poor compliance. Hence studies of correlations of BP declines with measures of compliance is somewhat like "comparing apples to oranges." A great deal of excitement has been engendered recently by the development of monitors that can be installed in the cap of a dispensing vial and register date and time whenever the cap is removed and a pill presumably withdrawn. Again, however, we are dealing primarily with a memory device for the patient who cannot remember when he or she took the last pill from the vial and how many were in it, so that this device does not seem to me to be anything more than a sophisticated and expensive form of pill counting.

Improvement in compliance can be accomplished by the various simple educational methods previously discussed. Additional strategies include reminder packaging but one study reported by Becker et al.[4] failed to show a difference when patients were given their medication in a special blister package with the time and date for each administration printed on the blister, as compared to the control group who received their medication in the standard medical vial. One study that employed self-monitoring of BP by the patients is reported to have raised compliance rates from 65% to 81%. Dunbar-Jacob et al. mentioned several studies that investigated specific educational strategies. Thus, Moriskey et al. found that counseling plus family support worked better than family support alone.[5] Kirscht et al. compared distribution of printed messages, nurse phone calls, self-monitoring of BP, and instruction by a self-identified support person. Only the latter two approaches—the nurse phone call and the instruction by the support person—had a significant impact on compliance, raising it to over 90% in these two groups.[6] Also mentioned by Dunbar-Jacob et al. is a study by Nessman[7] involving group therapy in which a group led by both a physician and nurse for a 90-minute instruction session weekly for 8 weeks showed significantly improved compliance as compared to its control group. Such involved strategies obviously are time-consuming, expensive, and hardly practical for the busy practitioner but they may have their value in specific therapeutic programs for hypertension. In effect, the aforementioned large-scale cooperative clinical trials used strategies of this type to keep their patients in therapy, and of course such programs have been in use for many years for other diseases requiring patient education such as diabetes. At the very least, these studies should encourage the individual physician to give or otherwise provide counseling to his or her individual patients.

Compliance has its roots in behavior and the changes that can be produced in the patient's attention and care of his or her hypertension by behavioral methods. It seems that providers interested in behavioral therapy would be well advised to employ their talents and time to working with patients with strategies to improve compliance rather than continued attempts to substitute relaxation, biofeedback, and related techniques, for effective pharmacological treatment. In this respect, and as summarized by Dunbar-Jacob et al.,[3] there is considerable need for carefully designed and controlled studies testing out various methods for this purpose. An interesting recent study with this goal is reported by McLane et al.[8] who derived a five-variable composite that includes: number of chronic illnesses, amount of time spent by physician with patient, patients' household support, family history of hypertension, and effect of hypertension on work and home activities. This composite served to identify potentially noncompliant patients and thus establish strategies to improve their compliance.

REFERENCES

1. Haynes RB, Improving patient compliance in the management of hypertension. In: Kaplan N, Ram CV, eds. *Individualized Therapy of Hypertension.* New York: Marcel Dekker, Inc; 1995:257-273.
2. Traub YM, McDonald RH Jr, Shapiro AP. Patient characteristics and their influence on therapy and its outcome in hypertension of the elderly. *Cardiology.* 1988; 75:45-55.
3. Dunbar-Jacob J, Dwyer K, Dunning EJ. Compliance with antihypertensive regimen: A review of the research in the 1980s. *Ann Behav Med.* 1991;13:31-39.
4. Becker LA, Glanz K, Sobel E, et al. A randomized trial of special packaging of antihypertensive medications. *J Family Pract.* 1986;22:357-361.
5. Moriskey DE, Levine DM, Green LW, et al. Five-year blood pressure control and mortality following health education for hypertensive patients. *Am J Publ Health.* 1983;73:153-162.
6. Kirscht JP, Kirscht JL, Rosenstock IM. A test of interventions to increase adherence to hypertensive medical regimens. *Health Educ Q.* 1981;8:261-272.
7. Nessman DG, Carnahan JE, Nugent CA. Increasing compliance: Patient-operated hypertension groups. *Arch Intern Med.* 1980;140:1427-1430.
8. McLane CG, Zyzanski SJ, Flocke SA. Factors associated with medication noncompliance in rural elderly hypertensive patients. *Am J Hypertens.* 1995;8:206-209.

8

Summary, Conclusions, and Future Goals

As implied in earlier chapters, my years of study of hypertension and hypertensive disease have led me into a variety of physiologic, biochemical, and clinical fields. A knowledge of epidemiology has been mandatory and the preventive aspects of illness have increasingly required my attention. The social and cultural impacts on hypertension have been noted. I have delved deeply into pharmacology, both basic and clinical, to understand the course and treatment of hypertension. Throughout all of this, I have maintained an abiding interest in the psychological and behavioral aspects of hypertensive disease, and my insights into this aspect of the disorder have been woven into my understanding of hypertension in an integral way. Sir George Pickering described hypertension as a continuum of BP measurements arranged in a normal distribution curve, wherein beyond a certain level, to the right side of the curve, individuals were labeled as hypertensive. Interspersed with this curve were persons with certain specific diseases, usually renal or endocrine, which deviated from the distribution curve and were specific entities that manifested high BP and its consequences. Irving Page provided the Mosaic Theory on which much of my thinking has been based, namely that essential hypertension as a clinical entity is not caused by any specific disorder, or failure but by an interlacing series of physiologic events that integrate with each other, and consequent to various checks and balances, can eventuate in hypertension. Guyton brilliantly theorized about the hemodynamics of hypertension and demonstrated the circumstances whereby any single mechanism can at one time be pressor and at another, depressor, depending on counterbalancing events. My thinking also leans heavily on the concept of disease developed by the late I. Arthur Mirsky, one of my major mentors, who believed that disease was the end result of a "chain of relevant biopsychosocial events." Mirsky applied this concept primarily to his studies of peptic ulcer, but it has equal pertinence to hypertension, and to me has been an intellectually and heuristically gratifying framework in which to study this disease. To appreciate this chain of relevant circumstances which lead to the disease, Mirsky argued that one has to understand the predisposition one individual has as compared to another to the given ailment; the precipitation, or onset, of the disease at one point in time rather than another; and the perpetuation of the disease rather than its resolution. Page's Mosaic Theory provides the mechanisms for each of these three influences and among these mechanisms psychological and behavioral events play at times a major role, and often a minor role, but probably never an exclusive role, as some investigators in the field have proposed.

Our approach to the question of the role of the stress produced by psychological influences on BP is based on the phenomenon of variability which we have discussed in detail earlier. Reactivity of BP to stimuli is one of the sources of variability. When it is pressor, it is considered to be a factor in precipitating and perpetuating hypertension; ethnic and genetic factors are thought to influence predisposition to these pressor responses. When reactivity is depressor, it is considered to be ameliorative and therapeutic and again can be considered in the context of the "three Ps." Much of the research on stress in hypertension has been devoted to elucidating these sequences, with the goal of defining the population that will become hypertensive from the impact of behavioral and psychological stimuli on the one hand, and the type and nature of stimuli which are evocative of these reactions, either pressor of depressor. Yet, although pursuit of the "Reactivity Hypothesis" has supported now several generations of investigators, including ourselves, and yielded a vast amount of fascinating data, the etiological role of such perturbations of the BP in the development of hypertension has not been resolved. To be sure, there are animal experiments in which at least transient elevations of BP have been produced from reactivity, but such efforts do not result in models that can compete with those produced by renal and endocrine manipulations and are most effective when superimposed on some predisposing condition that in itself might eventually produce hypertension. This is evident even in the now well-known, probably genetic, model of spontaneous hypertension in the rat, which can be brought on earlier and more severely with stress.

In summation, our conclusion at the present time is that reactivity is a subset of variability. If it has a precipitating outcome, it is a product of a quantitative impact rather than a qualitative one. The individual's genetic makeup or an acquired condition or disease (e.g., renal, adrenal, circulatory) may supply some degree of predisposition, but the reactivity is not the root cause of the hypertension. Where the individual resides on Pickering's distribution curve in regard to the development of clinical hypertension is primarily a function of original genetic status, and although the behavioral impact may at times be sufficient to be the precipitating factor, it is quite unpredictable and almost impossible to prevent. In my own considerable experience with hypertensive patients of all ages, types, and stages, I am convinced that I have seen and cared for many in whom the impact of the behavioral stress has been an important precipitating or perpetuating factor, but I am unable to provide hard data to convince myself or others of these sequences in the same fashion as I can with someone with renal artery stenosis or an adrenal gland tumor. At the same time, I have seen many patients with equally profound psychological and behavioral events affecting their lives that have not influenced the outcome of their disease other than producing transient elevations of BP. Similarly, the converse of the pressor response, the tendency for BP to fall with relaxation, biofeedback, reassurance, sleep, and the other influences we have discussed earlier is a fascinating phenomenon—or *epiphenomenon* as we have labeled it—but not a technique that can replace the potent and mechanism-directed pharmacological agents which we currently have available.

If we accept the concept that the etiology of hypertension is multifactorial with intertwining aspects of predisposition, precipitation, and precipitation then we can further propose how psychological and behavioral factors may impact in the quantitative fashion we have proposed. First, however, a brief recapitulation of theories of etiology is in order, both to summarize what we have said earlier, as well as to set the background for our further remarks about stress, psychological influences, and behavioral impact.

ETIOLOGICAL MECHANISMS IN HYPERTENSION

Hypertension is a disease that can be understood as a distortion of the physiologic mechanisms that ordinarily maintain BP at normal levels, as a first step to delivery of oxygen to peripheral tissues and organs. Cardiac output and peripheral resistance of the arterial blood vessels determine the BP and regulate the flow of blood to the periphery. Many factors influence these two basic functions but homeostatic regulatory mechanisms maintain BP at a relatively constant level by an elaborate feedback system. When cardiac output is raised and resistance does not fall, BP will rise. Conversely, change in the opposite direction will result in hypotension, while similarly if circulating volume rises and the kidney cannot handle the extra load, then output will rise and BP will become elevated. A whole series of events can occur resulting in such seemingly disparate situations as that seen in people with marked heart failure where cardiac output is very low, resistance is very high and BP in fact is low. Reducing resistance, or "unloading," in such a situation may actually cause BP to rise and improve cardiac function.

Theories of the etiology of essential hypertension have derived from the fact that there are certain known disease states in which hypertension is an inevitable development and with these models, investigators have sought the "Holy Grail" of single causation. Thus, there are those who would propose that the kidney is the major culprit because of its inability to handle sodium properly and hence fluid and sodium accumulate and hypertension develops. Other unitarians argue that a disturbance in the elaboration of renin or other pressor agents from the kidney, or conversely the failure of certain depressor agents (such as prostaglandin or kallikrein, or a renal medullary substance) to be present in adequate amounts, are the culprits. Another school would have us believe that disturbance in the ANS, and hence norepinephrine production, release or disposition, is the major cause and leads to increased peripheral resistance and/or increased cardiac output. Some of my colleagues in behavioral medicine have argued that stress through its effect on central adrenergic mechanisms is the prime etiologic mechanism in development of hypertension and certainly work cited earlier on midbrain mechanisms that can cause elevation of BP following acute and chronic stimulation of various parts of the brain would provide arguments for such a sequence. However, we should again point out that most theorists end up with a variant of the Mosaic Theory that Dr. Irving Page proposed a generation ago, although they put varying emphasis on different parts of the mosaic, and the "trigger points" in it. In fact, one can start at most any point in the homeostatic cycle and describe a feedback or failure of feedback system that can result in BP elevation. One needs only to have a model of the hemodynamic system, either an old-fashioned one such as we all used in physiology laboratories many years ago or a computer model such as Guyton developed, to demonstrate these possibilities and linkages.

Thus, the physiologic determinants of hypertension derive from a set of complex regulatory mechanisms that operate to maintain a relatively constant and adaptive relationship between the circulating fluid volume (i.e., cardiac output) and the space in which it circulates (i.e., peripheral resistance). An event that causes one mechanism to be unduly affected, as for instance isotonic exercise or other physical or psychological stress that increases cardiac output, results in feedbacks that cause vasodilatation and lower peripheral resistance. Failure of adequate vasodilation to occur, will result in a rise in BP, a sequence that may pertain to some essential hypertensives. The development of hypertension thus can depend on the failure and eventual breakdown of one or more loops of the feedback system and "single causation" becomes untenable even in those instances in which hypertension is referred to as "secondary" to another specific disease, in contrast to "primary" or essential (idiopathic) hypertension.

We can, however, view a number of the situations in which secondary hypertensions develop as instances in which autonomous control of one of the mechanisms develops (i.e., the stimulus is no longer under feedback control). Thus, the individual who has a pheochromocytoma has an autonomous source of norepinephrine that continually discharges and can cause both increased cardiac output and increased peripheral resistance. The patient with primary aldosteronism has a tumor that autonomously secretes mineralocorticoid and initially causes increased circulating volume and probably eventually increased peripheral resistance. Renal artery stenosis produces an ischemic kidney that autonomously stimulates the RAS rather than only in response to physiologic needs and can produce a permanent secondary hypertension. Renal parenchymal disease (i.e., chronic glomerulonephritis) eventuates in effect in an autonomous retention of salt and water with resultant overexpansion of circulating volume and rise in BP. Even these seemingly single causes must however be considered multifactorial because although the appropriate physiologic feedback systems cannot "turn off" the stimulus, adjustments such as decreased circulating volume in pheochromocytoma and renal "escape" in primary aldosteronism do attempt to correct the system and are usually "overwhelmed" by the persistent stimulus. Sometimes these adjustments are at least temporarily sufficient and certainly they can be taken advantage of in properly designed pharmacologic treatment. For instance, the patient with glomerulonephritis will have a fall in his or her renin activity; this encourages more "space for circulation" while reduction of sodium intake and judicious use of diuretics will further thwart this "autonomously sodium-retaining" kidney.

In primary (essential) hypertension, we are dealing with a situation in which we are unaware of which mechanisms in the system have failed. It is probable that they are multiple and it is in their elucidation that the factors of predisposition, precipitation, and perpetuation need further consideration and in which the psychological, behavioral, and social determinants play particularly significant roles.

BEHAVIORAL ETIOLOGICAL MECHANISMS

Some behavioral data, particularly those that have been previously cited as arising from epidemiological or disastrous events that seemingly led to hypertension, could be interpreted as evidence for a "pure pathogenic cascade" that affects the ANS and results in prolonged sympathetic hyperactivity (and perhaps some aspect of vagal inhibition) with resultant permanent hypertension. Using our discussion of failed feedback loops and "autonomous" control, one could thus interpret a situation in which stress is overwhelming as an instance when CNS and ANS mechanisms have become "autonomous" and the feedback checks and balances have become nonoperative. However, the sequences that are most appealing to us require a predisposition, either genetic or acquired, followed by precipitation and perpetuation as a consequence of "a chain of relevant psychological, socio-cultural and physical events" again using Mirsky's terminology. As mentioned earlier, Folkow, in his studies in spontaneously hypertensive rats, showed an enhanced central autonomic discharge that leads to an exaggerated cardiovascular response even before the rat's BP becomes elevated,[1] and proposed the following sequence:

1. Stress.
2. Genetically determined autonomic hyperactivity (or responsivity).
3. Intermittent rise in BP with elevated cardiac output.
4. Structural changes in resistance vessels.
5. Permanent hypertension.

In fact, there are a fairly significant group of studies in man of such sequences. These go back to Eich[2,3] and include the work of Julius and Schorck[4] showing that a large number, ranging perhaps from one third to two thirds of so-called borderline hypertensives, are high cardiac output hypertensives, who have been shown by Esler et al. to have high catechols and high renins.[5] Presumably, these patients "convert" when they eventually become "permanent hypertensives," to a normal output, high resistance set of hemodynamics. What is not known is the time frame for such changes. Eich's studies used a 5-year interval between observations, but it may occur sooner, or it may not occur at all because we see individuals who continue to show apparent cardiac hyperresponsivity for many years.

One rather interesting and unique study reported by Safar and his colleagues suggests a relationship between personality and hypertensive hemodynamics in a fashion that relates to our comments about perceptive changes as a consequence of the hypertension.[6] This group did Rorschach testing on patients with "borderline" hypertension and those with fixed hypertension and noted that change in hemodynamic pattern from high cardiac output to high peripheral resistance correlated with change in behavior from patterns in which anxiety and tension were high, to patterns displaying characteristics described as introspective, withdrawn and less expressive, the latter essentially a description of the so-called "hypertensive personality."

NEUROPHYSIOLOGIC SEQUENCE

The CNS pathways and mechanisms reacting to stress and leading to BP elevation are increasingly yielding to neurophysiologic investigation. The pattern of the hemodynamic response may be a consequence of the specific peripheral mediator (e.g., norepinephrine or epinephrine) but some studies have indicated that the cardiovascular adjustments may be exquisitely specific to different behaviors. Smith,[7] and Cohen and Obrist[8] reviewed this evidence and Zanchetti and coworkers[9] provided important data. For instance, their studies indicate that cats preparing to fight (agonistic behavior) display vasoconstriction and diminution of cardiac output, whereas during defensive behavior involving movement, increase in cardiac output and increase of muscle blood flow develop. Conditioning procedures involving these different types of behavior apparently also will produce these varying patterns. Hilton[10] suggested that the repertoire of basic response patterns in fact may be limited and that these cardiovascular basic patterns interreact when the behavior involves several of the activities, such as protective movements, exercise, and escape.

As outlined in an earlier chapter, pertinent to the development and study of models of hypertension related to stress are data available from the animal studies of Reis and his colleagues[11] who have produced neurogenic hypertension by lesions in the nucleus tractus solitarius (NTS) in the medulla. Such lesions abolish the baroreceptor reflexes and result in a labile hypertension. He and his colleagues[12] noted that classical conditioning of cats with bilateral lesions of the NTS results in a pressor response that is fives times greater than that obtained in similarly conditioned controls, which provides another example of predisposition, this time within the brain itself, which makes the animal more prone to precipitation of hypertension with appropriate stress.

SUMMATION OF ETIOLOGICAL SEQUENCES

Folkow's concept is remarkably similar to the paradigm which Mirsky proposed and offers a framework for future research. In Folkow's most recent writings he further defined the sequence of events that result in primary (essential) hypertension as the following:[13]

1. Polygenetically transferred predisposition, which varies among individuals and is reflected in animal studies by the different strains of rats, for instance, which have a tendency to hypertension.
2. Environmental factors which influence and reinforce the genetic tendency and include for instance sodium intake and psychoemotional influences.
3. Secondary adjustments which are initiated early in life and are reinforcing, or stabilizing, or counteracting. These adjustments are affected by positive feedback, and resetting or ineffectiveness of negative feedback.

Hypertension then ensues as a consequence of the balance of these components. Clearly, this is another way of stating the "three Ps" which Mirsky hypothesized and which we have used as a theme. Folkow's sequence is quite compatible with the idea that the outcome of the environmental effects on the genetic predisposition leading to the peripheral adjustments that are evidenced as the cardiac and resistance changes eventuating in hypertension, result from quantitative rather than qualitative impact. In other words, if the system is stressed frequently enough, even by events that are not necessarily traumatic, breakdown of compensating mechanisms can occur. In this respect, Folkow urged further research on the negative feedbacks that tend to counter pressor events and lower BP, as for instance the renomedullary substances that Muirhead studied for many years[14] and more recently have been relatively neglected.

THE REACTIVITY HYPOTHESES: DOES IT NEED FURTHER RESEARCH?

We have argued earlier that the pursuit of the reactivity hypothesis as an explanation for the development of hypertension has been underway now for many years without any consistent outcomes or "breakthroughs." We would submit that this theme has become exhausted and sterile and further explanations derived from studies of greater or lessor pressor responses to the vast variety of stimuli, both in the laboratory and in real life, will not be forthcoming. Similar thoughts have been expressed separately by Julius and his collaborators[15,16] and by Thomas Pickering et al.[17] Although Matthews et al.[18] have published a prospective study in a modestly sized group of children and their parents suggesting that BP changes to mental stress predicted future risk of hypertension over a period of 6 years, the amount of variance was quite small when corrected for a variety of factors, including the initial BP while development of actual hypertension in the group was minimal. Most revealing, is a recent report by Carroll et al.,[19] based on the Whitehall II study of 1000 civil servants in London who were followed for 4 to 7 years ($M = 4.9$) after screening and the administration of several stressful tests, and were then restudied. The sample came from a population of more than 10,000 persons, but women and anyone with a BP over 160/100 mm Hg, or receiving antihypertensive agents were eliminated. One of every four men who were eligible were chosen randomly for the study and follow-up. At follow-up, they noted minimal predictability of basal BP based on reactivity (1% for systolic and less than that for diastolic) although initial SBP and DBP were predictive of the follow-up BP variance at a level of 30% to 35%. The authors concluded that "measurement of reactivity is not a useful clinical index of the course of future BP." Although with the controversy about the "hyperreactivity hypothesis," the issue cannot be easily settled by this study, the often contradictory findings that have preceded it and the fact that it is perhaps the first large-scale study of the relationship of this nature causes me to view it with reasonable confidence that we are perhaps getting to the resolution of the matter. *The best predictor is the initial baseline pressure!*

Convincing further evidence of the role of the initial BP in determining predictability comes from the long term study of tracking of BP by Berenson and his colleagues. In a recent paper by Bao et al.,[20] the data from their Bogalusa study, which has now tracked BP from childhood to adulthood, were reported. In individuals now 20 to 31 years of age, prevalence of clinically diagnosed hypertension was much higher in subjects whose childhood BP was in the top quintile: 3.6 times as high in SBP and 2.6 times as high in DBP, compared to subjects in every other quintile. Of the 116 subjects who developed hypertension (of 1,505 studied) by this early adult age, 48% and 41% had elevated childhood systolic and diastolic hypertension, respectively. They conclude that elevated BP levels persist over time and progress to early adult hypertension and that repeated measurements of BP early in life improve the prediction of adult hypertension. My conclusion is that one does not have to measure reactivity to predict an eventual hypertensive outcome; *one only has to measure BP!* Pressor responses need not be aggravated in a particular group in order to have long-term impact but perhaps play a role when they are repetitive and corrective adjustments breakdown as suggested by Folkow.

SUGGESTED FURTHER RESEARCH

A question about reactivity that has always puzzled me is the implied distinction between "good and bad" cardiovascular reactivity. Thus, isotonic exercise with increased cardiac output is "good" for cardiovascular fitness, whereas isometric exercise, which increases peripheral resistance is considered "bad." On the other hand, pressor responses resulting from emotional stimuli are generally always considered "bad" even though some are cardiac reactions (output) and some are vascular reactions (peripheral resistance). Appropriate exercise thus is "good"; emotional stress is "bad" and can lead to hypertensive disease, or so the argument goes. In fact exercise is even encouraged to "relieve stress" and as pointed out in chapter 4, may have important nonpharmacologic therapeutic value in some hypertensive patients.

If one approaches this dichotomy from the quantitative, rather than the qualitative view, it makes more sense. Repetitive challenge of the negative feedback systems may reach a point with exercise as well as with noxious stimuli of emotional origin where the outcome is counterproductive. Similar mechanisms are involved in the production of the response and its counterbalancing with both types of stimulation. In fact, in some instances a cardiac response to exercise may be the counterbalance to a vascular response to an emotional stimulus. This seems to me a fertile field for future reactivity research, namely and simply, the pressor reactivity to a given emotional stimulus before, during, and after a physical exercise session, while for a "chronic model" we can study the well-conditioned athlete undergoing both the physical and emotional stress of a highly competitive game or race confrontation.

Another suggestion for further research if we are to get away from the continual search for meaningful pressor responses, is to devise means of studying the failure of depressor compensation. How to do this is as yet an enigma, but our increasing knowledge of various circulating and cellular molecules may be the direction in which we can head. Still another prospect for the future of pressor and depressor research may be in the emerging ability to study actual brain function with different stimuli through positron emission tonography (PET) scanning, which should show further methodological progress in the coming years. With such techniques, we may be able to work out the pathways between different stimuli and the neurological wiring of their responses and perhaps answer questions about whether certain stimuli are indeed more specific, pressor or depressor, than others or to what extent the responses are generalized.

Folkow[13] proposed another heuristic device as shown in Fig. 8.1. This is a schematic outline of the hierarchical organization and control of function in which Level III represents the area of local control (hemodynamics) at which most investigation has centered. More elucidation is needed at Levels I and II to understand precipitation, whereas current work at Levels IV and V may help to unravel the questions of secondary adjustment or perpetuation. The latter area poses a question that has long puzzled me, namely why an elevated BP actually causes the consequences that ensue from this elevation. If Sir George Pickering is correct, and developing hypertension is merely moving to the right on the normal distribution curve, the actual change is relatively small. Moreover, the damage is not always a correlate of the height of the pressure. Rabbits for instance have pressures that are only about 70 to 75 mm Hg and deteriorate at levels of 100 to 100 mm Hg, which in the rat and in man are harmless, whereas giraffes tolerate pressures of 200 to 250 mm Hg. Our present simple explanation is a strictly mechanical one and we use analogies such as the pipe or garden hose that is burst or stretched by a higher level of pressure than it was built to contain. Yet is this enough to account for hypertension as a risk factor for atherosclerosis and myocardial infarction, cardiac enlargement, renal damage, and cerebral thrombosis that are clearly derived from BP which moves to the right of Pickering's curve? Is it really something as simple as the need for the "pump" (the heart) to enlarge, which then "wears out" because it is working harder? Does the higher pressure "drive" cholesterol into the arterial wall? Does the pressure do something related to its height which affects the coagulation cascade?

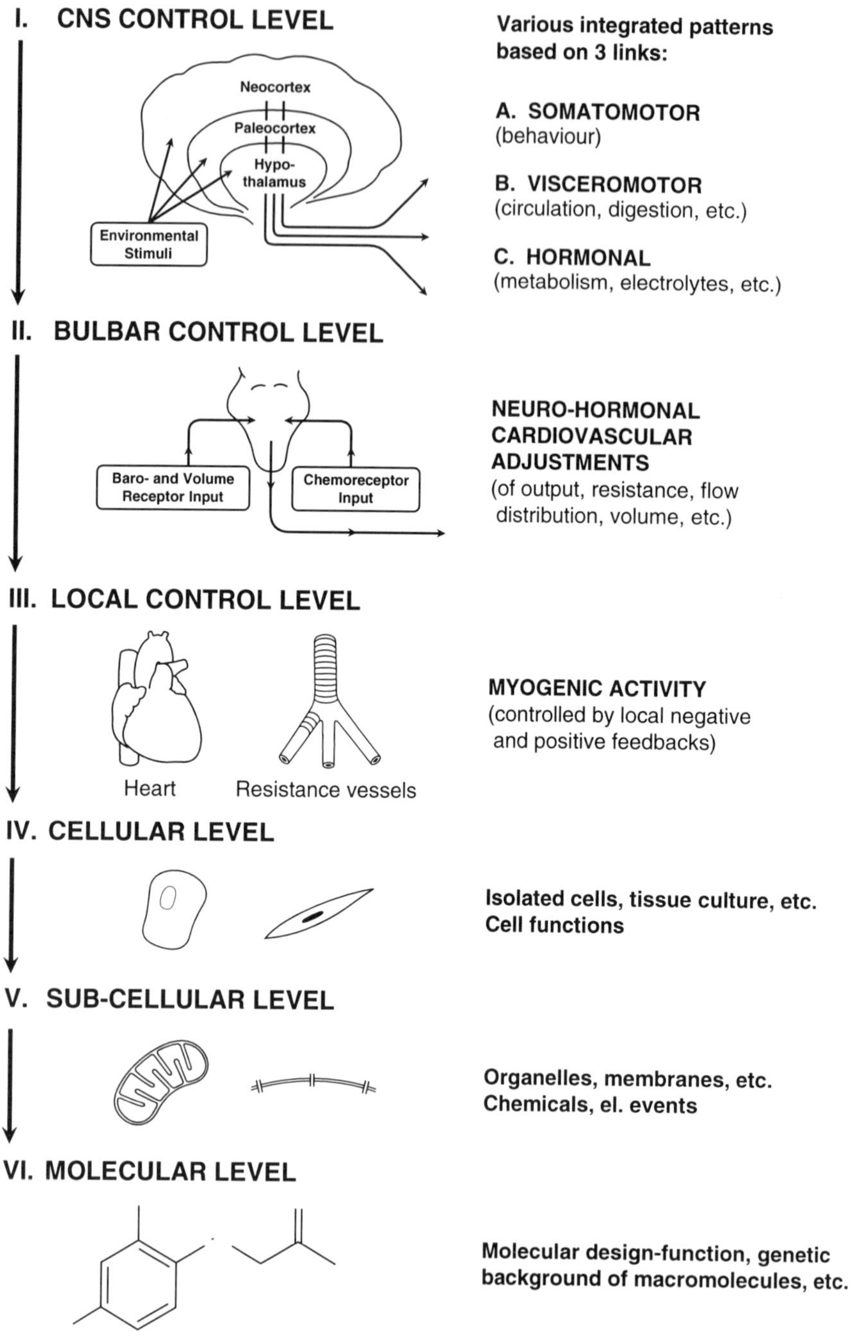

FIG. 8.1. Schematic outline of the six main levels of hierarchical organization and control in higher organisms, where the cardiovascular system at Level III represents the organ systems in the body (from Folkow, B. *J. Hypertension* 1995;13:5–18.).

These are questions that need to be approached at Levels V and VI and some progress is being made as for instance in recent studies of the effect of angiotensin II on molecular substances that influence vascular hypertrophy and on the damage that may be done to endothelium by deficiencies related to the nitric oxide (NO) system. As a clinician, dealing with the mechanical explanations (although very much part of our rational for treatment and by and large productive), I am impressed by the many patients who fail to progress or deteriorate despite "poor BP control" and the occasional patient who does poorly in spite of "good control." Because we know that most patients have a variable BP and are not usually at the level of pressure we perceive on our examination, we make assumptions that the total BP over time—what has been called the hyperbaric impact—is the culprit but we do not have the data to confirm this and will not until and unless we can develop simple and tolerable devices that will permit continuous monitoring for long periods of time. Such studies would then have to be performed with and without therapy, which would be impractical and probably unethical. A better approach is the molecular one to determine what factors cause the injury during long-term adjustment to a modest elevation of BP. And with this approach, the aforementioned shift of focus, which Folkow and others have discussed, of examining the failure of negative feedback systems, at all six levels of Folkow's schema, should be an area of future concentration.

The emerging data concerning endothelial-derived nitric oxide (NO) is particularly exciting in regard to the molecular consequences of hypertension. Not only does NO contribute to vasodilation but it also may inhibit cell growth and thus its deficiency may enhance medial hypertrophy. Pertinent to the understanding of CNS mechanisms, NO has been shown to decrease central sympathetic outflow and to elicit decreases in BP and HR within the NTS. Nitric oxide synthetases (NOS) are involved in the production of NO and their inhibition in the CNS results in elevation of BP. The RAS has also been shown to be affected by endogenous NO which can inhibit the release of renin and thus affect angiotensin release. NOS inhibition can raise BP while angiotensin converting enzyme (ACE) inhibitors and angiotensin receptor blocking agents seem to prevent this elevation indicating a role for activation of the RAS in the production of increased BP by NOS inhibition.[21-23]

An exciting approach that combines the behavioral aspects of cardiovascular disease to molecular events is represented by the recent work of Williams and his colleagues who have studied the vasodilator responses of the coronary arteries in cymologus monkeys to psychosocial stress.[24,25] They have shown that the vasodilator response is impaired by chronic stress through an impairment of endothelium-derived relaxing factor (EDRF). They suggest that such data may have considerable importance in providing molecular mechanisms for understanding stress effects in CAD and, we would add, for further understanding of vasoconstriction from the impact of behavioral events on BP control.

As further goals for the future of research in hypertension are at least two additional and important areas that concern themselves with behavior and both are components of the pharmacological aspects of hypertension. We have earlier discussed in detail the problems of compliance with medication in a disease that at least in our present state of knowledge is not subject to "cure," but requires a lifelong commitment to therapy. This is, as we have described, a psychosocial problem that demands the use of a variety of educational techniques and productive research in this area is to be encouraged. The other is the further expansion and continuation of studies such as the ones we, as well as others, have initiated, on the behavioral consequences of hypertension and the effects of different drugs and classes of drugs on these behaviors. These will be studies primarily at Levels I and II of Folkow's paradigm but will include aspects of perpetuation and adjustment from Levels V and VI.

CODA

A few concluding comments, derived from the historical record of research in hypertension and our own involvement in both research and clinical areas, are in order. Research in hypertension has largely been concerned with the hemodynamics of BP control. In effect, the observations of the Reverend Stephen Hales were hemodynamic and most of our clinical efforts at BP control have dealt with its hemodynamic parameters. The vast literature on stress and hypertension and the revelations related to reactivity and variability are primarily concerned with hemodynamic changes. Sir George Pickering's argument that BP represents a normal distribution with hypertension as the "right-hand side of the curve" relates to hemodynamics with prevalence defined by where one places the dividing line. Page's Mosaic Theory provides a concept that is a heuristically valuable framework for research in etiology and mechanisms. But we have moved on now into an era in which further effort at understanding mechanisms and future gains in control of this disorder will come from information derived from molecular biology. This is not to say that we should discard the hemodynamic data so carefully accumulated in the past, but rather to learn to integrate it with present day and future insights. Folkow warned quite passionately and appropriately about the dangers of reductionism and the "disregard for the immensely complex integrative mechanisms which are the hallmark of higher organisms"[13] and again the Mosaic Theory provides this concept.

My text has been written primarily to elucidate the progress and status of behavioral factors in hypertension and their contribution through stress and psychological influences to this mosaic. In our own work and formulations, we have tried to be protean in this regard so that the impact of hypertension derived from renal mechanisms on the psyche of a given patient has been as important in understanding management as the impact of the office visit on the patient with "White Coat Hypertension." Continued exploration of the behavioral parameters remains an important area for research and clinical application but it is time to move on from the aforementioned hemodynamic studies of stress effects on BP per se that have so flooded the field. The newer molecular observations cited previously need exploration, in particular as they pertain to CNS mechanisms and integration. In so doing, we can maintain a place for the behaviorally interested clinician and the biologically oriented psychologist in the further understanding of Mirsky's "chain of relevant psychosocial biological circumstances" which predispose, precipitate, and perpetuate hypertensive disease.

REFERENCES

1. Folkow B, Hallback M, Lundgren Y, Sivertsson R, Weiss L. Importance of adaptive changes in vascular design for establishment of primary hypertension, studied in man and in spontaneously hypertensive rats. *Circ Res.* 1973;32(Suppl 1):2-B.
2. Eich RH, Peters RJ, Cuddy RP, Smulyan H, Lyons R. The hemodynamics in labile hypertension. *Am Heart J.* 1962;63:188-195.
3. Eich RH, Cuddy RP, Smulyan H, Lyons RH. Hemodynamics in labile hypertension (a follow-up study). *Circ.* 1966;34:299-307.
4. Julius S, Schork MA. Borderline hypertension—a critical review. *J Chronic Dis.* 1971;17:397-404.
5. Esler M, Zweifler A, Randall O, Julius S, DeQuattro V. The determinants of plasma renin activity in essential hypertension. *Ann Intern Med.* 1978;88:746-752.
6. Safar ME, Kamienecka HA, Dimitru VM, Levenson JA, Pauleau NF. Hemodynamic factors and Rorschach testing in borderline and sustained hypertension. *Psychosom Med.* 1978;40:620-630.
7. Smith AO. Reflex and central mechanisms involved in the control of the heart and circulation. *Ann Review of Physiology.* 1974;36:93-123.
8. Cohen DH, Obrist PA. Interactions between behavior and the cardiovascular system. *Circ Res.* 1975;37:693-706.
9. Zanchetti A, Baccelli G, Mancia G. Cardiovascular effects of emotional behavior. In: Bartorelli C, Zanchetti A, eds. *Cardiovascular Regulation in Health and Disease.* Milano: Instituto di Recherche Cardiovasculari; 1970:17-32.
10. Hilton SM. Ways of viewing the central nervous control of the circulation—old and new. *Brain Res.* 1975;87:213-219.
11. Reis DJ, Doba N. The central nervous system and neurogenic hypertension. *Progress in Cardiovascular Disease.* 1974;27:51-71.
12. Nathan MA, Tucker LW, Severini WH, Reis DJ. Enhancement of conditioned arterial pressure responses in cats after brainstem lesions. *Science.* 1978;201:71-73.
13. Folkow B. Integration of hypertension research in the era of molecular biology: G.W. Pickering memorial lecture (Dublin 1994). *J Hypertension.* 1995;13:5-18.
14. Cowley AW Jr. Evolution of the medullipin concept of blood pressure control: a tribute to Eric Muirhead. *J Hypertension.* 1994;12(suppl 10):S25-S34.
15. Weder AB, Julius S. Behavior, blood pressure variability, and hypertension. *Psychosom Med.* 1985;47:406-414.
16. Julius S, Weder AB, Hinderleiter AL. Does behaviorally induced blood pressure lead to hypertension? In: Matthews KA, Weiss SM, Detre T, Dembrowski TM, Falkner B, Manuck SB, Williams RR, eds. *Handbook of Stress, Reactivity, and Cardiovascular Disease.* New York: Wiley; 1989:71-81.
17. Pickering TG, Gerin W. Cardiovascular reactivity in the laboratory and the role of behavioral factors in hypertension: a critical review. *Ann Behav Med.* 1990;12:3-16.
18. Matthews KA, Wood KL, Allen MT. Cardiovascular reactivity to stress predicts future blood presssure status. *Hypertension.* 1993;22:479-485.
19. Carroll D, Smith GD, Sheffield D, Shipley MJ, Marmot MG. Pressor reactions to psychological stress and prediction of future blood pressure: data from the Whitehall II study. *BMJ.* 1995;310:771-776.
20. Bao W, Threefoot SA, Srinivasan SR, Berenson GS. Essential hypertension predicted by tracking of elevated blood pressure from childhood to adulthood: the Bogalusa Heart Study. *Am J Hyp.* 1995;8:657-665.

21. Kanagy NL, Webb PC. Cyclic GMP-independent effects of nitric oxide in the vasculature: a role in the pathogenesis of hypertension. *High Blood Pressure Research.* 1995;3:7-15.
22. Luscher TF. The endothelium in hypertension: bystander, target or mediator? *J Hypertension.* 1994;12(suppl 10):S105-S116.
23. Jover B, Herizi A, Ventre F, Dupont M, Mimran A. Sodium and angiotensin in hypertension induced by long-term nitric oxide blockade. *Hypertension.* 1993;21:944-948.
24. Williams JK, Vita JA, Manuck SB, Selwyn AP, Kaplan JR. Psychosocial factors impair vascular responses of coronary arteries. *Circ.* 1991;84:2146-2153.
25. Williams JK, Kaplan JR, Manuck SB. Effects of psychosocial stress on endothelium-mediated dilation of atherosclerotic arteries in cynomolgus monkeys. *J Clin Invest.* 1993;92:1819-1823.

Author Index

Numbers in parenthesis are reference numbers and indicate that the author's work is referred to although the name is not cited in the text. Numbers in italic show the page on which the complete reference is given.

F

G

H

I

J

Subject Index

D